VASECTOMY:
Current Research In Male Sterilization

Papers by
Frederick J. Ziegler, J.C. Smith, John M. Beazley,
Anne Roe, Nathan Hershey, Pauline Jackson, Moni
Nag, Helen Wolfers, D. Urquhart-Hay, I.F. Potts,
Philip M. Alderman, Donald Young, George Watts,
Andrew S. Ferber, K.H. Moon, P. Rumke, H.J.
Roberts, J. Robert Rinker, Benjamin L. Pagovich,
A.M. Rakha, K.A. Norberg, J.D. Skinner, Howard
G. Hanley, R.C.B. Pugh, Manuel Fernandes, Edward
E. Steinhardt, K.C. Mehta, K.L. Macmillan et al.

MSS Information Corporation
655 Madison Avenue, New York, N. Y. 10021

Library of Congress Cataloging in Publication Data
Main entry under title:

Vasectomy.

   1. Vasectomy--Addresses, essays, lectures.
I. Ziegler, Frederick J. [DNLM: 1. Sterilization,
Sexual--Collected works. 2. Vas Deferens--Surgery--
Collected works. WJ 780 V332 1973]
[RD571.V37 1973]   613.9'42'08   72-13573
ISBN 0-8422-7097-3

TABLE OF CONTENTS

Vasectomy as a Contraceptive Measure   9

Psychosocial Response to Vasectomy . . . . Ziegler,
Rodgers and Prentiss   10

Vasectomy, Ovulation Suppressors
and Sexual Behavior . . . . Ziegler and Rodgers   30

Semen Examination after Vasectomy . . . . Smith   55

Voluntary Sterilization . . . . Beazley and Fraser   56

Vasectomy: Research Proposal . . . . Roe   61

Abortion and Sterilization: Status
of the Law in Mid-1970. . . . . Hershey   62

A Male Sterilization Clinic. . . . . Jackson, Phillips,
Prosser, Jones, Tindall, Crosby,
Cooke, McGarry and Rees   66

Vasectomy and Adverse
Psychological Reactions . . . . .Ziegler   73

Is Sterilization the Answer? . . . . Nag   76

Psychological Aspects of Vasectomy. . . . . .Wolfers   77

Voluntary Sterilization in the Male . . . . . .Urquhart-Hay   86

Medico-Legal Implications of Vasectomy . . . . Potts   92

Vasectomy for Voluntary
Male Sterilization. Alderman   93

Medical Aspects of Vasectomy   95

Vasectomy for Contraception . . . . .Young   96

Vasectomy for Sterilization. . . . . Watts   97

Men with Vasectomies: A Study
of Medical, Sexual and Psychosocial
Changes. . . . . Ferber, Tietze and Lewit   98

Lacate Dehydrogenase Isozyme
Patterns in Pre- and Postvasectomy
Seminal Plasma . . . . Moon and Bunge   111

Sperm-Agglutinating Autoantibodies
in Relation to Male Infertility . . . . Rümke   115

Voluntary Sterilization in the Male . . . . Roberts   119

Spermagglutinin Formation in Male
Rats by Subcutaneously Injected Syngeneic
Epididymal Spermatozoa and by Vasoligation
or Vasectomy . . . . Rümke and Titus   120

Delayed Thrombophlebitis and Systemic
  Complications after Vasectomy: Possible
    Role of Diabetogenic Hyperinsulinism . . . . Roberts   131

A Statistical Study of Unilateral
  Prophylactic Vasectomy in the
    Prevention of Epididymitis: 1029
      Cases . . . . Rinker, Hancock and Henderson   145

Subcutaneous Inguinal Vasectomy
  in Conjunction with Abdominal
    Prostatectomy . . Pagovich, Horowitz and Weinberg   146

Hormonal Physiology of Vasectomy **149**

Pituitary Gonadotrophins (Follicle-
  Stimulating Hormone and Interstitial
    Cell-Stimulating Hormone) and Seminal
      Vesicular Fructose after Long-Term
        Vasectomy in Bulls . . . . . . Rakha and Igboeli   150

Adrenergic Innervation of the Male
  Reproductive Ducts in Some Mammals.
    II. Effects of Vasectomy and
      Castration . . . . . Norberg, Risley and Ungerstedt   153

Some Effects of Unilateral Cryptorchism
  and Vasectomy on Sexual Development
    of the Pubescent Ram and
      Bull . . . . Skinner and Rowson   159

Reversal of Vasectomy **173**

Vasectomy for Voluntary Male Sterilization . . . . Hanley   174

Spontaneous Recanalization of the
  Divided Vas Deferens . . . . Pugh and Hanley   182

Vasovasostomy: Improved Microsurgical
  Technique . . . . Fernandes, Shah and Draper   190

Vasovasostomy: A Simplified Technique . . . Steinhardt   194

Splinted and Nonsplinted Vasovasostomy:
  Experimental Study . . . . Moon and Bunge   198

Bilateral Spontaneous Reanastomosis of
  the Ductus Deferens . . . . .Bunge   204

A Simple Technique of Reanastomosis
  after Vasectomy . . . . Mehta and Ramani   205

Veterinary Vasectomy. **209**

Gonadal and Extragonadal Sperm Reserves
  after Unilateral Vasoligation in
    Rabbits . . . Macmillan, Desjardins, Kirton and Hafs   210

CREDITS AND ACKNOWLEDGEMENTS

Alderman, Philip M., "Vasectomy for Voluntary Male Sterilization," *The Lancet*, September 23, 1968, pp. 1137-1138.

Beazley, John M.; and W.J. Fraser, "Voluntary Sterilization," *The Lancet*, September 6, 1969, p. 531.

Bunge, R.G., "Bilateral Spontaneous Reanastomosis of the Ductus Deferens," *The Journal of Urology*, 1968, 100:762.

Ferber, Andrew S.; Christopher Tietze; and Sarah Lewit, "Men with Vasectomies: A Study of Medical, Sexual, and Psychosocial Changes," *Psychosomatic Medicine*, 1967, 29:354-366.

Fernandes, Manuel; Kanu N. Shah; and John W. Draper, "Vasovasostomy: Improved Microsurgical Technique," *The Journal of Urology*, 1968, 100:763-766.

Hanley, Howard G., "Vasectomy for Voluntary Male Sterilization," *The Lancet*, July 27, 1968, p. 207.

Hershey, Nathan, "Abortion and Sterilization: Status of the Law in Mid-1970," *American Journal of Nursing*, 1970, 70:1926-1927.

Jackson, Pauline; Betson Phillips; Elizabeth Prosser; H.O. Jones; V.R. Tindall; D.L. Crosby; I.D. Cooke; J.M. McGarry; and R.W. Rees, "A Male Sterilization Clinic," *British Medical Journal*, 1970, 4:295-297.

Macmillan, K.L.; C. Desjardins; K.T. Kirton; and H.D. Hafs, "Gonadal and Extragonadal Sperm Reserves after Unilateral Vasoligation in Rabbits," *Fertility and Sterility*, 1968, 19:982-990.

Mehta, K.C.; and P.S. Ramani, "A Simple Technique of Reanastomosis after Vasectomy," *British Journal of Urology*, 1970, 42:340-343.

Moon, K.H.; and R.G. Bunge, "Lacate Dehydrogenase Isozyme Patterns in Pre- and Postvasectomy Seminal Plasma," *Investigative Urology*, 1968, 6:223-226.

Moon, K.H.; and R.G. Bunge, "Splinted and Nonsplinted Vasovasostomy: Experimental Study," *Investigative Urology*, 1967, 5:155-160.

Nag, Moni, "Is Sterilization the Answer?," *Science*, 1970, 168:62.

Norberg, K.-A.; Paul L. Risley; and U. Ungerstedt, "Adrenergic Innervation of the Male Reproductive Ducts in Some Mammals. II. Effects of Vasectomy and Castration," *Experientia*, 1967, 23:392-397.

Pagovich, Benjamin L.; Marcel I. Horowitz; and Sidney R. Weinberg, "Subcutaneous Inguinal Vasectomy in Conjunction with Abdominal Prostatectomy," *The Journal of Urology*, 1968, 100:52-53.

Potts, I.F., "Medico-Legal Implications of Vasectomy," *British Journal of Urology*, 1970, 42:737-738.

Pugh, R.C.B.; and Howard G. Hanley, "Spontaneous Recanalization of the Divided Vas Deferens," *British Journal of Urology*, 1969, 41: 340-347.

Rakha, A.M.; and G. Igboeli, "Pituitary Gonadotrophins (Follicle-Stimulating Hormone and Interstitial Cell-Stimulating Hormone) and Seminal Vesicular Fructose after Long-Term Vasectomy in Bulls," *Fertility and Sterility*, 1971, 22:581-583.

Rinker, J. Robert; Carl V. Hancock; and William D. Henderson, "A Statistical Study of Unilateral Prophylactic Vasectomy in the Prevention of Epididymitis: 1029 Cases," *The Journal of Urology*, 1970, 104:303.

Roberts, H.J., "Delayed Thrombophlebitis and Systemic Complications after Vasectomy: Possible Role of Diabetogenic Hyperinsulinism," *Journal of the Geriatrics Society*, 1968, 16:267-280.

Roberts, H.J., "Voluntary Sterilization in the Male," *British Medical Journal*, August 17, 1968, p. 434.

Roe, Anne, "Vasectomy: Research Proposal," *Science*, 1970, 168:1523-1525.

Rümke, Ph., "Sperm-Agglutinating Autoantibodies in Relation to Male Infertility," *Proceedings of the Royal Society of Medicine*, 1968, 61:275-277.

Rümke, Ph.; and M. Titus, "Spermagglutinin Formation in Male Rats by Subcutaneously Injected Syngeneic Epididymal Spermatozoa and by Vasoligation or Vasectomy," *Journal of Reproduction and Fertility*, 1970, 21:69-79.

Skinner, J.D.; and L.E.A. Rowson, "Some Effects of Unilateral Cryptochism and Vasectomy on Sexual Development of the Pubescent Ram and Bull," *Journal of Endocrinology*, 1968, 42:311-321.

Smith, J.C., "Semen Examinations after Vasectomy," *The Lancet*, January 2, 1971, p. 38.

Steinhardt, Edward E., "Vasovasostomy: A Simplified Technique," *Henry Ford Hospital Medical Journal*, 1969, 17:67-70.

Urquhart-Hay, D., "Voluntary Sterilization in the Male," *New Zealand Medical Journal*, 1970, 71:230-232.

Watts, George, "Vasectomy for Sterilization," *British Medical Journal*, April 12, 1969, p. 119.

Wolfers, Helen, "Psychological Aspects of Vasectomy," *British Medical Journal*, 1970, 4:297-300.

Young, Donald, "Vasectomy for Contraception," *British Medical Journal*, November 11, 1967, pp. 354-355.

Ziegler, Frederick J., "Vasectomy and Adverse Psychological Reactions," *Annals of Internal Medicine*, 1970, 73:853.

Ziegler, Frederick J.; David A. Rodgers; and Robert J. Prentiss, "Psychosocial Response to Vasectomy," *Archives of General Psychiatry*, 1969, 21:46-54.

Ziegler, Frederick J.; and David A. Rodgers, "Vasectomy, Ovulation Suppressors, and Sexual Behavior," *Journal of Sexual Research*, 1968, 4:169-194.

PREFACE

During the past decade vasectomy has been used successfully on a large scale as a means of human population control, particularly in India. Its obvious advantages are that it is effective, inexpensive, quick, and requires no subsequent care or concern on the part of the patient.

This new collection summarizes recent research on vasectomy. Clinical evaluations and populational studies are first presented, followed by physiological, social and forensic aspects of this contraceptive technique. The medical aspects covered include resultant psychosocial and sexual changes, patterns in pre- and postvasectomy seminal plasma, sperm-agglutinating autoantibodies in relation to infertility, and systemic complications following vasectomy. The hormonal physiology of vasectomy is considered in a separate section. As documented in the text, vasectomy can be reversed by medical procedures and will sometimes reverse by spontaneous anastomosis; new surgical techniques are also presented, as well as the veterinary practice of vasectomy.

Vasectomy as a Contraceptive Measure

Psychosocial Response to Vasectomy

Fredrick J. Ziegler, MD
David A. Rodgers, PhD
Robert J. Prentiss, MD

MEN electing vasectomy for contraception and their wives were studied with interviews, psychological tests, and questionnaires over a four-year period beginning prior to surgery. They were compared to ovulation-suppression-using couples. After four years, the two groups did not differ significantly in frequency of intercourse or other sexual behavior, changes in sexual problems, emotional adjustment, or changes in marital satisfaction. Consistent with earlier evaluations, the vasectomy men showed evidence of a counteractive reaction to threats to masculinity with an increase in masculinity-confirming behavior. The study procedures probably attenuated adverse psychological reactions. Other men not interviewed showed psychological test evidence of emotional upset following vasectomy. Suggestions are made concerning selection of appropriate subjects for the operation, and for other contraception methods, and concerning appropriate procedures to reduce risk of negative postvasectomy emotional reactions.

Voluntary male sterilization, vasectomy, has not been an unusual method of contraception in recent years. In 1960, approximately 7% of husbands of fertile wives in the western United States had obtained a vasectomy, whereas the national incidence was approximately 2%.[1] Aside from its intended function of surgically induced sterility, no adverse physiologic effects of vasectomy have been demonstrated or seriously proposed. A number of reports, however, have addressed themselves to the possibility of alterations in psychological functioning after vasectomy. In various interview and questionnaire follow-up studies conducted in the United States, Europe, and Asia, over 90% of the subjects and their wives in all the reported studies expressed satisfaction with vasectomy as a contraceptive procedure.[2-7] Some of these reports, however, and other reports[8-10] indicate that psychological complications following vasectomy are fairly common. The discrepancy in reported satisfaction of the subjects with vasectomy on the one hand, and evidence of psychological problems on the other, was pointed up by Dandekar,[2] who found that 92% of 1,191 men were "favorable to vasectomy" after the operation, but that 53% reported "weakened sexual desire." Lee[7] reported general enthusiasm for vasectomy in Korea, but in the same paper reported a group of 20 postvasectomy "sterilization neuroses" attributed to presumed confusion of sterilization with castration. Ferber et al[3] reported that, of 73 men who agreed to be interviewed after they had been helped by the Human Betterment Association to obtain a vasectomy, there was general satisfaction with vasectomy as a contraceptive procedure, but six told the psychiatric resident interviewers that it was a personal sacrifice to have had the vasectomy. These authors felt that the results were ultimately generally good and concluded that:

These men and their friends and relatives hold stereotyped attitudes equating vasectomy with being castrated and made inferior, and . . . the good results indicate adequate coping with these psychological factors by a large majority of the respondents.[3]

Johnson[9] reported that in 83 male patients hospitalized in a Veterans Administration Psychiatric Hospital at some time following a vasectomy, the vasectomy often seemed to have played a significant role in their disturbed psychological functioning and family

11

relationships. This seemed particularly so in 11 instances. Parker et al reported to the American Psychiatric Association in 1965,[10] that "the effects of sterilization result in major psychologic upheaval frequently enough to warrant thorough reevaluation of the medical and psychiatric reasons supporting the procedure."

None of the reports of other investigators to date has, however, been "controlled" in the sense that there was a suitable comparison group, and none has been done using a longitudinal or prospective design. Since 1960, the present authors and their associates have collaborated in conducting a longitudinal or prospective study, with a comparison group, in order to assess changes in psychological functioning and in marital relations following vasectomy. The present report primarily concerns data from 42 couples who were systematically assessed by structured psychiatric interviews, psychological testing, and questionnaire reports over a four-year period beginning prior to having vasectomies performed by private practicing urologists. A comparison group of 42 couples was studied during this same time period, beginning just before being given first prescriptions for ovulation suppression pills by private practicing gynecologists. The details of research design, findings, and our formulations of the studies through the two-year follow-up period have been previously reported.[11] The vasectomy group, with few exceptions noted below, consistently attributed only favorable changes to vasectomy, blaming other life circumstances for any adverse changes in their emotional functioning or their family situation. As a group, however, the men and their wives showed somewhat more psychological pathology at that time than did the women and their husbands in the pill-taking group, both as assessed by changes in psychological testing and by ratings of mental status from the protocols of the psychiatric interviews. At that time, the vasectomy couples rated their

Table 1.—Actuarial Characteristics of Subjects

	Pill		Vasectomy	
	Men	Women	Men	Women
Age	30.9	28.0	33.1	30.6
Age, 1st intercourse	17.7	19.5	18.0	19.3
Education	13.9	13.0	13.8	13.0
Religion				
Protestant	16	15	23	24
Catholic	2	3	9	7
Jewish	0	0	3	3
Other, none	4	4	2	3
Number of subjects	22		37	
Years married	7.7		9.4	
Number of children	2.5		3.1	
Income				
Under $5,000	1		1	
$5,000-$10,000	12		16	
$10,000-$15,000	8		14	
$15,000-$20,000	1		4	
Over $20,000	0		2	

own marriages significantly less enthusiastically than did the comparison group couples. The study then seemed to replicate the reports of others that men and their wives generally express enthusiasm for vasectomy after they have turned to this contraceptive method, but that evidence of adverse psychological changes is demonstrable if one looks for it. We ascribed these paradoxical findings to "dissonance reduction,"[12] in which persons in some situations tend to reassure themselves by focusing primarily on favorable considerations, ignoring or rationalizing contradictory evidence. We concluded:

The data suggests that the operation is responded to as though it had demasculinizing potential, with a result that the behavior of the man after vasectomy is more likely to be scrutinized by himself and others for evidence of unmasculine features. Behavior questioned as possibly unmasculine is anxiety-provoking and tends to be eliminated, narrowing the range of acceptable behaviors on a highly individualized basis reflecting each person's circumstances and interpretation of "unmasculine." In some instances, the result is a salutary decrease in immature and indecisive behavior, with improvement in occupational, parental, and husband role enactments. In other and perhaps more characteristic instances, the decreased flexibility reduces personal effectiveness, heightens personal anxiety, and abrades marital harmony and the satisfactions of the wife.

In the present report we will consider these same couples from the vantage point of additional information from three- and four-year follow-up evaluations. Thirty-seven couples of the vasectomy group completed the four-year study program. One couple of the original 42 could not be traced, one couple was divorced and the wife could not be traced, one man was killed in an auto accident, one man and one wife of another subject refused to complete the final questionnaire. Thirty-seven couples of the ovulation-suppressor group also completed the four-year study program. Eleven of the ovulation-suppression group had stopped pills in order to have a planned pregnancy; this group tended to be younger and in other respects was not comparable to the vasectomy couples or to the remaining pill using couples. Of the remaining couples, 14 continued on ovulation suppressors for the duration of the study, while 8 discontinued the pills with no intention of returning to them for contraception and with no intention of becoming pregnant. In the present comparisons with the vasectomy couples, the ovulation-suppressor group will consist of these 14 "continuous" and 8 "discontinuous" couples. The remaining four pill group couples will, like the pregnancy group, be ignored because of difficulty classifying them: two of these women discontinued the pills following hysterectomy; one discontinued on medical advice after a breast lump was discovered; and one couple discontinued the pills, had an unplanned pregnancy, and then returned to the pills so that they could not be considered either "continuous" or "discontinuous." Results of the studies of the ovulation-suppressor sample as a whole, with emphasis on several consistent differences that were demonstrable between the "continuous" and the "discontinuous" couples, have been previously reported.[13] Details will not be repeated here.

Selected actuarial characteristics of the 37 vasectomy couples and of the 22 comparison (combined "continuous" and "discontinuous") ovulation-suppressor-using couples are shown in Table 1. The primary difference between the groups is that the vasectomy couples are slightly older and have slightly larger families. Otherwise the two groups are reasonably comparable.

Results

Satisfaction With Vasectomy as a Contraceptive Procedure.—After vasectomy, one man and his wife and the wife of another subject stated that they would not again choose vasectomy as their contraceptive method. Additionally, one man and his wife, two wives of other subjects, and one other male subject stated that they had considered reversal of the vasectomy operation because of religious convictions or (in the case of the couple) because they felt that vasectomy had adversely affected their sexual relationship. Two additional wives considered that vasectomy had adversely affected their sexual relationships. A total of 10 of 74 subjects, then, somewhat more than in reports of other investigators, had direct complaints about vasectomy as a contraceptive method. More wives expressed doubts about it than did the men themselves.

Satisfaction With Marriage.—In contrast to the way these couples rated their marriages at two-year follow-up, there were no significant differences between the vasectomy couples and the comparison group at the end of four years (Table 2). The men in the ovulation-suppressor group tended to rate their marriages somewhat more highly than did the men in the vasectomy group, but they had also done so initially and the change was not significant.

Interview and Questionnaire Evaluation of Psychiatric Status.—Questions in the structured interviews and questionnaires relating to psychiatric symptoms were evaluated for each subject in the study by three psychiatric residents independently. Differences in their ratings were readily reconciled in a joint conference (Table 3). There

15

were no significant differences when the mean ratings were compared across groups. The husbands of the women who discontinued ovulation suppressors showed the most negative changes and, because of this, 55% of the husbands in the pill group showed some negative change, compared to 38% of the husbands in the vasectomy group. Comparison of the women in the two groups indicated essentially identical results for both groups. The differences were not statistically significant.

Psychological Test Findings.—The subjects were given the California Psychological Inventory (CPI) initially and at two-year and three-year follow-up. They were given the Minnesota Multiphasic Personality Inventory (MMPI) at six-month and three-year follow-up. Estimated MMPI profiles were determined from the CPI data[14] for the initial and two-year follow-up periods. Changes of the vasectomy group from preoperative to three years on the standard MMPI and CPI scales did not exceed chance levels. The profiles for each subject were clinically assessed for significant emotional changes. Four of the men in the vasectomy group showed rather marked increase of anxiety and depression. Seven showed corresponding decrease of these

Table 2.—Marital Satisfaction*

	Pill (N=22)		Vasectomy (N=37)	
	Men	Women	Men	Women
Initial	1.2	1.0	1.1	1.1
2 years	1.3	1.0	1.0	0.8
4 years	1.2	1.1	1.0	1.2

Mean of ratings from −1 to +2.

Table 3.—Clinical Ratings of Emotional Upset*

	Men			Women		
	Initial	2 yr	4 yr	Initial	2 yr	4 yr
Pill (N=22)	1.1	1.3	1.5	1.7	1.6	1.6
Vasectomy (N=37)	1.2	1.2	1.3	1.7	1.6	1.6

*4 is the highest degree of upset.

symptoms, but this decrease seemed often to be counterbalanced by marked increase in general defensiveness and rigidity. When subjects were rated as worse or better on testing, with a marked increase in either emotional upset or defensiveness being considered a negative change, 12 of the 37 vasectomy men showed negative change and only two showed positive change. These frequencies did not differ significantly from the husbands of the combined pill groups, however, six of whom showed negative changes and two, positive changes out of 22 subjects. Corresponding figures for the wives were one positive and seven negative changes in the vasectomy group and three positive and four negative changes in the pill group, the groups again not differing significantly. Other relevant testing results have been previously reported.[11,13,15]

Sexual Behavior.—Relatively complete analyses of the data concerning sexual behavior of the subjects have been previously reported.[16,17] Relevant findings were as follows:

Frequency of Intercourse.—The vasectomy group initially reported a lower frequency of intercourse than did the pill group, but at the end of four years, there was no significant differences between the two total group averages (Fig 1). Comparison of these data to other norms suggested that an initially depressed rate of intercourse tended to increase with effective, nonintrusive contraception.

Use of Noncoital (Oral and Manual) Orgastic Techniques.—At the four-year follow-up, more than three fourths of the subjects reported that they occasionally practiced oral or manual genital orgastic stimulation of their partner. Roughly one half had initially reported using these techniques, at which time a number of the subjects rationalized them as substitute sex behavior because of inadequate contraception. Since the subjects' reported use of these techniques however, did not decrease after effective contraception, and additional subjects re-

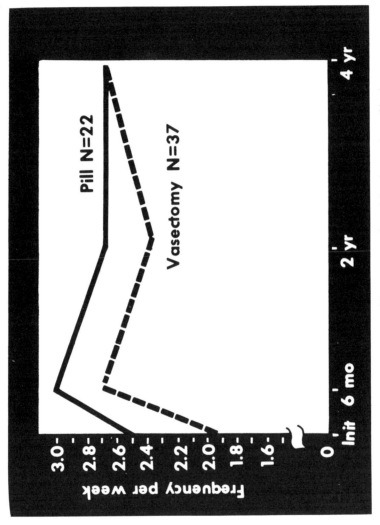

Fig 1.—Stated frequency of intercourse, male and female reports combined.

18

Fig 2.—Frequency of intercourse by groups differing in sexual problems.

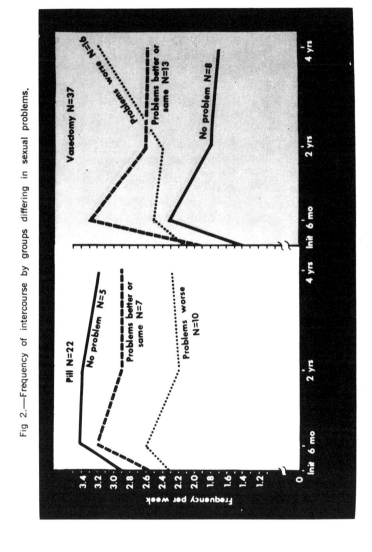

ported using them, it seemed clear that they are employed because of intrinsic interest and not because of fear of pregnancy or as a contraceptive substitute. There were no notable differences across groups.

Extramarital Sexual Relations.—In general, there was no convincing evidence that effective contraception increased probability of extramarital sexual relationships. Over all, 63% of the men and 85% of the women denied ever having had extramarital relationships, and approximately 19% of the men and 7% of the women were actively involved in such affairs at any one time, both before and after effective contraception.

Frigidity.—Reported frigidity of the female subjects did not differ significantly between the two groups and was not changed appreciably after vasectomy or after use of ovulation suppressors. Effective contraception, then, did not apparently have any notable effect on female frigidity; and vasectomy would not seem to be indicated as an attempted remedy for such a marital problem.

Impotence and Premature Ejaculation.—Sixteen of the 37 men of the vasectomy group reported more problems with impotence, premature ejaculation, or sexual drive by the end of four years than preoperatively, 13 men reported that these problems were the same or better than they were preoperatively, and an additional 8 men reported no problems at all. Correspondingly, ten of the pill-group men reported more problems, 7 reported problems that were the same or better, and 5 reported no problems at all. Proportionately, then, there was no notable difference between the two groups. However, when each of these subgroups were examined for frequency of reported intercourse, an interesting difference became apparent (Fig 2). The husbands of the women using ovulation suppressors showed the expected relationship of highest rate of intercourse being associated with the fewest sexual problems, whereas the vasectomy group showed exactly the opposite relationship at the end of the study. Men whose sexual problems got worse after vasectomy reported the highest frequency of intercourse, whereas those who reported no sexual problems showed the lowest frequency of intercourse of any group in the study. We would usually expect men with impotence problems to reduce rather than to increase frequency of intercourse, and would expect men using effective contraception who have no problems with impotence to report relatively higher frequencies of intercourse—as was reported by the pill group. The unexpected reversal of frequencies reported by the vasectomy subgroups suggests to us the possibility that the men who had sexual problems after vasectomy tended to overcompensate by increasing rather than decreasing the frequency of intercourse. This is consistent with our previous inference that men have strong needs to deny any decrease in masculinity after vasectomy and that aspects of their behavior are often understandable as overcompensation for these needs.

The basis for these unusual relationships between sexual problems and frequency of intercourse was further assessed, as follows: The men in the vasectomy group were classified into three groups: (1) Those who reported both an increase in sexual problems and an increase in rate of intercourse by the end of the study (12 subjects); (2) all men who denied ever having any problems with impotence or premature ejaculation and whose rate of intercourse was lower at the end of the study than it had been previously (7 subjects); and (3) all other subjects (18 in number). The latter group consisted primarily but not entirely of men who reported a decrease in sexual problems during the study. These three groups were then compared on changes on the CPI *Do* (dominance) and *Re* (responsibility) scales, two scales that measure, respectively, a person's tendency to make demands on his environment and his tendency to assume the obligations imposed by his environment. These two scales are normally positively correlated

21

($r = +0.35$ for a sample of over 4,000 men and $+0.36$ for a sample of over 5,000 women, reported in the CPI Manual),[15] and tend to change in a positively correlated manner on test-retest comparisons. The change on each scale was determined for each subject between initial testing and three-year follow-up. For the subgroup that showed increase in both sexual problems and frequency of intercourse, these before and after changes on *Do* and *Re* correlated -0.37. For the subjects reporting no sexual problems and a decrease in frequency of intercourse, the correlation was -0.48. For the remaining subjects, who showed a more expected relationship between frequency of intercourse and sexual problems, $r = +0.67$, significantly different from both of the other groups ($P < 0.05$, by standard error of difference between z's). Seventy percent of the increased-problems increased-frequency group showed an increase on *Do* and a decrease on *Re*, indicating an increase in demandingness and a decrease in tendency to assume responsibilities. This compares to only 11% of the "remainder" group who showed a similar response. Similarly, 71% of the no-problems low-frequency group showed a decrease in both *Re* and *Do*, indicating a decrease in tendency both to make demands and to accept responsibility. This compares to 33% of the "remainder" group who showed such a response. Thus, both of the groups who reported an unusual relationship between sexual problems and frequency of intercourse showed deviant correlations and other test changes suggesting less willingness to assume responsibilities. Those who had an increase in sexual problems tended to become more demanding and those who reported no sexual problems tended to become less demanding and seemingly less involved generally in interpersonal relationships.

We interpret these test changes as supporting the inference that the increased-problems increased-frequency group reacted counteractively to their sexual problems by becoming more generally demanding and less compliant, or more "culturally masculine," as well as more demanding in their sexual relationship with their wives. That is, we infer that these men, when faced with physiologic evidence of impairment of masculine function, reacted by becoming more aggressive and assertive and less socially conforming, thus attempting confirmation of their masculinity by their social behavior as a way of denying loss of masculinity associated with impotence or other sexual problems. We infer that in the marriage situation and in the sexual relationship, these same men aggressively demanded more rather than less sexual activity than there had been in spite of their own apparent less adequate performance. Consistent with this inference is the fact that a higher percentage of the wives of these men had frigidity problems in spite of the higher frequency of intercourse than did the wives of either of the other groups (25% frigidity in this group of wives compared to 14% in the low-problem low-frequency group and 17% in the "remainder" group). We infer that the no-problems decreased-frequency group, which did not have their masculinity threatened by specific sexual problems, reacted to the operation or perhaps other unknown stresses by a degree of general disengagement from interpersonal relationships, including disengagement from sexual relationships with their wives.

At the end of four years then, there was no impressive evidence that couples after vasectomy, when studied in the manner which we have described, were psychologically worse off than a comparison group of couples if assessed by indicators of pathology or disturbance. There was indication that even four years after vasectomy, men were still concerned about any evidence of loss of masculinity and were attempting to compensate for it by an increase in the frequency of intercourse and other behavioral changes. To date, we have been unable to identify a group of men in the present study who were especially vulnerable to the psychological hazards of vasectomy. Different men showed different aspects of both positive and negative postoperative changes, apparently reflecting rather individualized ways of reacting. No group of significant size showed an identifiable consistent negative (or positive) response. Because of this we doubt the utility of reporting here the numerous additional subanalyses that have been done on this particular group of subjects in attempts to identify a "higher risk" or "lower risk" type of candidate for vasectomy.

Effect of Study on Postoperative Response.—Considering the general concern about psychological problems after vasectomy, in the reports cited above, it may seem surprising that these subjects did not show more gross changes in their postoperative psychological functioning. It has more and more become our conviction that these couples, initially well selected for having rational reasons for vasectomy and for having a stable family situation,[19] were buffered from notable adverse psychologic change after vasectomy by the extensive contact with the study team. In the more formal structured interviews with each subject (which became "open-ended" after the structured portion was finished), in the questionnaires, and in the miscellaneous telephone calls to the study couples from the investigators keeping track of their life situations, these men and their wives had considerable opportunity to clarify any possible questions in their minds about any aspect of vasectomy, as well as the opportunity to explore in significant detail their current life adjustment problems, concern about their sexual relationships, sexuality in general, etc. It seems to us that this relationship of the study team with the subjects probably aborted, or "defused," those psychologic complications which it was presumably designed to observe, describe, and clarify.

Corollary Study.—Evidence strongly supporting the point of view that the interviewing attenuated the psychological impact of vasectomy comes from another study we conducted prior to the present one, of 35 other men who obtained vasectomies from private practicing urologists. These men had no contact with the investigators, but were given a short questionnaire and the MMPI prior to vasectomy. They completed a follow-up questionnaire and a repeat MMPI (which were sent to them through the mail) 1 to 1½ years postoperatively.[20] Only one of these men reported that he would not have the operation again if the choice were still open; general enthusiasm was high, as was found in the other postoperative surveys cited above. However, in this study which collected minimal data without "feedback" and without contact with the investigators, most clinical MMPI scales were significantly elevated at follow-up as compared to the preoperative testing. Fifteen of the subjects were considered to show negative postoperative test changes, contrasting with two who were considered to show psychological improvement. We consider that this study (which was a prospective study without a comparison group) more accurately assesses the usual frequency and degree of psychological changes after vasectomy since medical contacts with these subjects more closely approximated usual medical practice. We therefore infer retrospectively that this group of subjects is more appropriate than the more intensively studied couples to examine for criteria that would be helpful to urologists in selection of patients for vasectomy. We found that the hypochondriacal scale (scale 1) of the MMPI significantly identified the unfavorable responders ($P < 0.02$ Wilcoxon Rank Sum Test), those with the highest scores being more prone to show subsequent negative changes. Additionally, five subjects who showed markedly adverse psychological changes after vasectomy were found to have had significantly higher preoperative scores on the masculine-feminine scale (scale 5) of the MMPI than did the subjects who did not respond

25

negatively $(P < 0.05$, Wilcoxon Rank Sum Test), suggesting that preoperatively this group may have had some doubt about their masculinity. On the questionnaire items, those subjects who had initially rated either their health or wife's health as less than excellent tended significantly postoperatively to change for the worse psychologically. These findings suggest that, ordinarily, hypochondriacal men or those who have doubts about their own masculine effectiveness would be poorer surgical risks, in terms of vulnerability to psychological reactions after vasectomy.

Comment

Our studies as well as others reported in the literature indicate that adverse psychological changes can occur in response to vasectomy. We interpret the evidence as indicating that vasectomy is reacted to by most subjects and their wives as if the operation had "demasculinizing potential," such that an increase in psychologic upset or in compensatory stereotyped masculine behavior or both is found in a high percentage of subjects. In the presently reported intensive study, severely adverse psychological changes were few, and, we infer, were largely aborted by the discussion with the investigators. The subjects were also undoubtedly rather effectively prescreened by the urologists who performed the operations. Nevertheless, even within this group, there is consistent evidence that a vasectomy can be a continuing challenge to a man's conception of himself. In a previous study, we have shown that two quite different cultural subgroups (college students and a Protestant church group) held derogatory attitudes toward couples who rely on vasectomy for contraception as contrasted to couples using ovulation suppression[1]; and we infer that such attitudes are widely prevalent in most cultural groups and are even held to some extent by the men who obtained vasectomy and by their wives. After a couple has selected vasectomy as a desirable contraceptive procedure for rational reasons that presumably outweigh their covert negative attitudes, full therapeutic discussion of their concerns and their reactions would theoretically be expected to modify their covert unfavorable attitudes, such that their vulnerability to the impact of negative cultural judgments and to psychological upset would be reduced. We infer that such reduction in vulnerability occurred in the present study. In any event, and especially if the foregoing inference is correct, the conclusion seems warranted that if a man, his wife, and a physician conclude that vasectomy is a desirable contraceptive method for the couple and if the couple has adequate opportunity to discuss all implications of the procedure with an informed person, the ultimate effect of vasectomy on psychological functioning and marital adjustment will, on the average, be comparable to the effect of electing ovulation suppression. We would suggest even more specific differential bases, however, for selecting couples for vasectomy as opposed to ovulation suppression or other contraceptive procedures. As we have noted,[9] some couples with identifiable characteristics apparently respond well to use of ovulation-suppressor contraceptives; and some couples, with other identifiable characteristics, discontinue ovulation suppression if it is once started, show adverse psychological changes, and often have further unwanted pregnancies. We suggest that couples in which the wife finds sexual relationships pleasurable and desirable, is able to assume responsibility in the family, is not subordinate to her husband socially or intellectually, is conscientious and responsible, and is able and willing to take responsibility for contraception, will find ovulation suppression or one of the "feminine" contraceptive methods such as an intrauterine device, diaphragm and jelly, etc, highly satisfactory either for spacing pregnancies or for more permanent contraception. We suggest that in families where the husband is more socially and intellectually effective and the wife is more subordinate, more unwilling to take responsibility for contraception, and less interested in sexual behavior generally, a masculine form of contraception will be more satisfactory. The husband may use condoms or the more risky method of withdrawal for the spacing of pregnancies and for more permanent contraception if the couple is willing to accept the small, but not negligible, risk of unwanted pregnancies. If completely effective and permanent contraception is desired by such couples, if the husband is not particularly hypochondriacal or concerned about the health of his wife or himself, and if the husband has no apparent doubts about his own masculinity, then vasectomy might well be the contraceptive procedure of choice, especially if covert concerns about it can be adequately discussed pre- and post-operatively. In summary, then, it seems to us that the results of these studies argue strongly for individualized contraceptive medical advice, that each procedure has its identifiable assets and hazards, and that vasectomy can be regarded as a desirable alternative under the conditions specified.

Supported primarily by Public Health Service Research grants MH 04479 and MH 13360 from the National Institutes of Mental Health. We wish to thank Sali Ann Kriegsman and Jane Qualls for their assistance on the study. The cooperation of urologists, Drs. R.M. Boughton, D.S. Brown, F.H. Carter, R.E. Delaval, J.C. Hayward, G.D. Howe, R.E. Lawton, E. LeDuc, V. Moore, S.B. Nuzie, R.T. Plumb, R.A. Pullman, and J.M. Whisenand, and gynecologists, Drs. K.E. Crippen, P.L. Martin, and S. H. Smith is gratefully acknowledged.

References

1. Campbell, A.A.: The Incidence of Operations that Prevent Conception, *Amer J Obstet Gynec* 89:694-700 (July 1) 1964.

2. Dandekar, K.: After-Effects of Vasectomy, *Artha Vijnana* (Gokhale Institute of Politics and Economics, Poona, India) 5:212-224 (Sept) 1963.

3. Ferber, A.A.; Tietze, C.; and Lewit, S.: Men with Vasectomies: A Study of Medical, Sexual, and Psychosocial Changes, *Psychosom Med* 29:354-366 (July-Aug) 1967.

4. Garrison, P.L., and Gamble, C.J.: Sexual Effects of Vasectomy, *JAMA* 144:293-295 (Sept 23) 1950.

5. Hauser, E.: Die Sterilisation des Mannes zur Verhütung von Schwangerschaften, *Praxis* 44:477-484 (May) 1955, and 44:500-506 (June) 1955.

6. Landis, J.T., and Poffenberger, T.: The Marital and Sexual Adjustment of 330 Couples who Chose Vasectomy as a Form of Birth Control. *J Marriage Family* 27:57-58 (Feb) 1965.

7. Lee, H.Y.: Studies on Vasectomy: III. Clinical Studies on the Influences of Vasectomy, *Korean J Urology* 7:11-29 (May) 1966.

8. Hinderer, M.: Über die Sterilisation des Mannes und ihre Auswirkungen, *Schweiz Arch Neurol Psychiat* 60:145-149, 1947.

9. Johnson, M.H.: Social and Psychological Effects of Vasectomy, *Amer J Psychiat* 121:482-486 (Nov) 1964.

10. Parker, J.B., Jr.: Hallock, H.L.: and Longstaff, J.P.: *Sequelae of Sterilization of Self or Marital Partner*, read before the meeting of the American Psychiatric Association, New York, May 1965.

11. Ziegler, F.J.: Rodgers, D.A.: and Kriegsman, S.A.: Effect of Vasectomy on Psychological Functioning, *Psychosom Med* 28:50-63 (Jan-Feb) 1966.

12. Festinger, L.: *A Theory of Cognitive Dissonance*, Stanford, Calif: Stanford University Press, 1962.

13. Ziegler, F.J., et al: Ovulation Suppressors, Psychological Functioning, and Marital Adjustment. *JAMA* 204:849-853 (June 3) 1968.

14. Rodgers, D.A.: Estimation of MMPI Profiles from CPI Data, *J Consult Psychol* 30:89 (Feb) 1966.

15. Rodgers, D.A., et al: Comparisons of Nine Contraceptive Procedures by Couples Changing to Vasectomy or Ovulation Suppression Medication. *J Sex Research* 1:87-96 (July) 1965.

16. Rodgers, D.A., and Ziegler, F.J.: Changes in Sexual Behavior Consequent to Use of Noncoital Procedures of Contraception, *Psychosom Med* 30:495-505 (Sept-Oct) 1968.

17. Ziegler, F.J., and Rodgers, D.A.: Vasectomy, Ovulation Suppressors, and Sexual Behavior. *J Sex Research* 4:169-193 (Aug) 1968.

18. Gough, H.G.: *Manual for the California Psychological Inventory*. Palo Alto, California: Consulting Psychologists Press, Inc., 1957.

19. Rodgers, D.A., et al: Sociopsychological Characteristics of Patients Obtaining Vasectomies from Urologists, *Marriage and Family Living* 25:331-335 (Aug) 1963.

20. Rodgers, D.A., et al: A Longitudinal Study of the Psycho-Social Effects of Vasectomy, *J Marriage Family* 27:59-64 (Feb) 1965.

21. Rodgers, D.A.: Ziegler, F.J.: and Levy, N.: Prevailing Cultural Attitudes About Vasectomy: A Possible Explanation of Postoperative Psychological Response, *Psychosom Med* 29:367-375 (July-Aug) 1967.

Vasectomy, Ovulation Suppressors, and Sexual Behavior

FREDERICK J. ZIEGLER and DAVID A. RODGERS

A number of writers (e.g., Tietze, 1952) have emphasized that effectiveness of a contraceptive method cannot be studied without reference to its acceptability by users. The converse is almost axiomatic, that acceptability is dependent in part upon assumed effectiveness. Acceptability is apparently much greater for those methods that are not directly related to the act of coitus (such as ovulation suppressing pills, intrauterine devices, vasectomy, and tubal ligation) than it is for methods used in direct relationship to intercourse (Polgar and Guttmacher, 1966). Coital contraceptive techniques (such as the condom, diaphragm, foam, withdrawal, or rhythm) emphasize the potential fertility of the partners, since their use is a constant reminder of the possibility of conception. Their less-than-perfect record of protection (Tietze, 1962) further reinforces the tendency to associate coitus with potential procreation. In contrast, the non-coital methods divorce pleasurable sexuality from the possibility of procreation, partially because they are essentially completely effective but primarily because they make continuous infertility—rather than potential fertility—the routine state for the user.

The possibility that conception might result could, consciously or unconsciously, motivate sexual behavior and contribute to sexual

This investigation was supported in part by research grant MH-04479 from the National Institute of Mental Health, Public Health Service, and was undertaken with the cooperation of urologists Drs. R. M. Boughton, D. W. Brown, F. H. Carter, R. E. Delaval, J. C. Hayward, G. D. Howe, R. E. Lawton, E. LeDuc, V. Moore, S B. Nuzie, R. T. Plumb, R J. Prentiss, R. A. Pullman, and J M. Whisenand; and gynecologists Drs. K. D. Crippen, P L. Martin, and S. H. Smith.

We gratefully acknowledge the assistance on this project of John Altrocchi, Ph.D., Sali Ann Kriegsman, Nissim Levy, Ph.D., Jeannine Ludwig, and Neil Whitworth, and express our appreciation to the numerous professional colleagues who have served as consultants.

Data processing has been greatly facilitated by access to the computer located at the University of California at San Diego.

Medication was supplied by G. D. Searle and Company, Chicago, Illinois, and Ortho Pharmaceutical Corporation, Raritan, New Jersey.

arousal and pleasure (Lehfeldt, 1959). From this point of view, the separation of sexual pleasure from reproduction, as with non-coital methods of contraception, would seem logically self-defeating. A contrasting contemporary point of view holds that fear of pregnancy and sexual pleasure exist in dynamic biological—but not psychological—counterpoint. Separation of the two, it is felt, could open a Pandora's Box of cultural problems ranging from almost universal infidelity and irresponsible hedonism, to a population crash and even eventual disappearance of those groups with unrestricted access to completely effective contraception. Although few data exist by which these points of view can be empirically evaluated, much effort in both the public and the private sectors of world economy is being directed toward achieving the goal of contraception without impairment of sexual pleasure. Empirical data concerning the effects of ovulation suppression and of vasectomy—two effective non-coital techniques—on sexual behavior may therefore be of some general interest.

PROCEDURE

The present data were collected in conjunction with a prospective study of the psychosocial consequences of vasectomy for contraception and of use of ovulation suppressing pills. Details of the study design have been described previously (Ziegler, et al., 1966). Data were obtained from couples referred by private practicing urologists, shortly before a vasectomy was performed on the husband, and by private practicing gynecologists, shortly before the wife began use of ovulation suppressing pills. Husband and wife were interviewed privately and sequentially by one investigator (FJZ) with no chance to compare responses between interviews. The interviews followed a standardized structured format designed to elicit relevant information which included a comprehensive sexual history. The data were recorded during the interviews. Each subject also completed extensive psychological testing which is not considered in the present report. Approximately four months after the vasectomy or the initial use of ovulation suppressors, each subject was asked to complete additional tests and a questionnaire that elicited information about sexual as well as other behavior. Between one and two years after the initial contact, each couple was again interviewed and tested. As in the first interview, the husband and wife were seen sequentially by the same person (FJZ), and the discussion followed a structured format. More complete data on parameters of sexual behavior, such as estimates of duration of intercourse and of duration of time from penetration to ejaculation, were elicited in the final interviews than in the initial ones.

Data reported in the present paper are derived from all couples who completed the overall study, who were married throughout the study, and who continued using the contraceptive of choice during the intervening period. These consisted of 41 couples utilizing vasectomy (designated the "V" group) and 23 couples relying on contraceptive pills (designated the "P" group). Since not all subjects provided complete answers to every question, frequencies reported in the tabulated data sometimes total less than these numbers of subjects. In the overall study, data were obtained from an additional vasectomy couple, but they had divorced before the second interview and are not included in the present report. Similarly, data not reported here were obtained in the overall study from 19 additional pill couples. Two of these did not complete follow-up studies; one had obtained a vasectomy and discontinued use of the pills; one was not married at time of initial assessment; one was divorced at time of final follow-up; and the remaining 14 had discontinued use of the pills. Of these 14, seven stated that they had discontinued pills because of desire for pregnancy, four because of side effects, two because of extraneous medical problems, and one because of infrequency of sexual relations.

As in nearly all such studies, the data collected denote subjective estimates reported retrospectively by the subjects—persons who were not alerted to the need for accurate observation during the behavior reported on, and who may have had personal reasons for wanting to distort the data. However, most respondents seemed interested in the study and generally cooperative, and the method of tandem interviewing employed, combined with initial lack of knowledge of the nature of the study or of the particular questions to be asked, probably prevented active collusion between husband and wife concerning the information given.

RESULTS

Actuarial characteristics of the sample at the beginning of the study are summarized in Table 1. They describe the subjects providing information and should not be interpreted to characterize the populations of subjects choosing the particular methods of contraception

TABLE 1

..tuarial Characteristics of Subjects at Beginning of Study

Characteristic	V Group				P Group			
	Husband		Wife		Husband		Wife	
	Mean	S.D.	Mean	S.D.	Mean	S.D.	Mean	S.D.
Age (Years)	33.3	5.7	30.5	5.9	29.3	6.4	26.1	6.0
Years married to present spouse	9.7	5.6	9.7	5.6	6.2	5.0	6.2	5.0
No. of children from present spouse	3.1	1.2	3.1	1.2	2.3	1.1	2.3	1.1
Years of education	13.7	2.5	12.9	2.0	13.5	1.6	12.8	1.6
Age at first orgasm	12.7	1.8	17.7	3.8	13.2	1.8	17.8	5.0
Age at first intercourse	17.6	3.3	19.1	4.0	17.3	3.2	18.9	1.9

	Per Cent of Subjects			
Experience causing first orgasm				
Intercourse	7	51	0	39
Petting	2	10	0	30
Masturbation	73	20	74	9
Dreams	12	2	26	4
Other	2	2	0	9
Omitted or?	2	15	0	9
Amount of premarital sex experience				
No experience or spouse only	17	63	9	78
1–10 partners	54	35	70	22
More than 10 partners	31	2	22	0
History of contraceptive failure with present spouse	49	49	48	48
Religion in which reared				
Protestant	44	61	78	70
Catholic	29	15	13	13
Jewish	7	10	0	0
None	20	15	9	17
Other	0	2	0	0
Present religious beliefs				
Protestant	66	68	65	70
Catholic	22	17	9	13
Jewish	7	7	0	0
None	2	5	26	17
Other	2	2	0	0
Present religious affiliation				
Protestant	44	54	48	61
Catholic	20	15	9	13
Jewish	5	2	0	0
None	32	27	43	26
Other	0	2	0	0

represented. That is, no attempt was made to obtain a representat. sampling of all couples choosing vasectomy or of all couples choosing pills. The sample is biased toward white Southern California couples seeking help from medical specialists rather than from general practitioners or non-medical sources, toward subjects who are willing and intellectually able to participate in a study involving extensive self-administered testing, and toward couples who are sufficiently concerned about family limitation to seek expert advice. These characteristics tend to limit the sample to middle or upper-middle class couples, primarily in the young adult age range.

Other papers have considered (Rodgers, *et al.*, 1963; Rodgers, *et al.*, Feb. 1965; Rodgers, *et al.*, July 1965; Ziegler, *et al.*, 1966) and will further consider, psychological aspects of using vasectomy or ovulation suppression for contraception. In the present report of the sexual histories elicited, data will be presented separately for the two groups, and if significant effects might be attributable to the specific contraceptive chosen, this will be indicated. In general, however, the focus will be on consequences of effective non-coital contraception, per se, and not on specific method used. Therefore, there has been no attempt to equate the two groups of subjects in the samples reported here. The following significant differences between the groups (Table 1) should be noted: the V group is somewhat older, on the average, than the P group (the differences in age of husband, age of wife, and years married are all significant, $p < .05$, by t-test), and the V group has significantly more children ($p < .01$, by t-test). Otherwise, the groups are of essentially similar socio-economic and psychological status (Ziegler, *et al.*, 1966).

Figure 1 summarizes information on reported frequency of intercourse prior to the operation or use of the pills. Table 2 summarizes husband-wife correlations for reported frequency and duration of intercourse and for preferred rates. In Figures 2 and 3, reported changes in frequency of intercourse during the first four-month interval, and from initial assessment to final follow-up are shown.

The relationship between rate of intercourse and age is shown in Figures 4 and 5. The rates shown are those reported at the final follow-up, when contraception was presumably considered effective and fear of pregnancy would not be an issue. Table 3 summarizes product-moment correlations between rate of intercourse and age variables, indicating levels of significant departure from zero. Table 4 shows

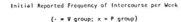

Initial Reported Frequency of Intercourse per Week

(· = V group; x = P group)

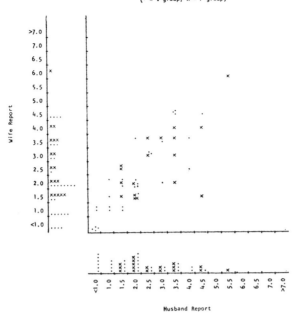

Husband Report

FIGURE 1

TABLE 2

Product Moment Correlations Between Husband and Wife Reports

	Group	
	P	V
Frequency of intercourse, initial interview.................	.66**	.88***
Frequency of intercourse, final interview...................	.79**	.83***
Husband's preferred rate, initial interview.................	.51*	.37*
Wife's preferred rate, initial interview.....................	.26	.54**
Husband's preferred rate, final interview..................	.45	.70***
Wife's preferred rate, final interview......................	.78**	.75***
Total duration of intercourse, final interview..............	− .17	.57***
Duration of penetration to ejaculation, final interview.......	.69**	.24

*, **, *** indicate p <.05, .01, and .001, respectively.

mean reported rates of intercourse at initial evaluation and at final follow-up, as well as estimates of duration of intercourse, obtained at follow-up. Only data from couples who provided adequate information about frequency at both the initial and the final evaluations

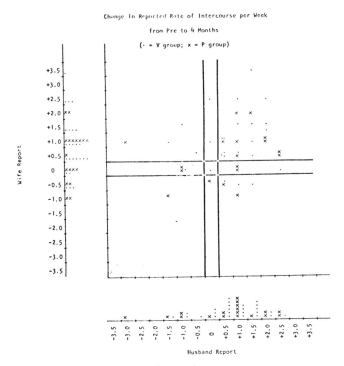

Change In Reported Rate of Intercourse per Week

from Pre to 4 Months

(· = V group; x = P group)

FIGURE 2

were included in Table 4, which therefore should reflect any changes that resulted from the increased certainty of contraceptive control. The initial rate of the V group is significantly lower than is that of the P group, as reported by the husband (p < .05). The same directional trend is apparent in the data from the wives, but does not reach statistical significance. The differences have essentially disappeared by final follow-up, however, since the V group shows a significant increase in frequency (p < .001 for husbands' reports, p < .01 for wives' reports, t-test). The P group fails to show a significant change.

Figures 6 and 7 show the discrepancy between preferred frequencies of intercourse and actual frequencies, according to the husbands and according to the wives, at initial interview and at final follow-up. At both the initial and the final interview, each subject stated his or her perception of actual frequency of intercourse, as well as his or her preferred frequency. These data thus provide a direct basis for classifying each subject as being satisfied with actual rate, unsatisfied (if preferred rate exceeds actual), or sated (if actual rate exceeds

36

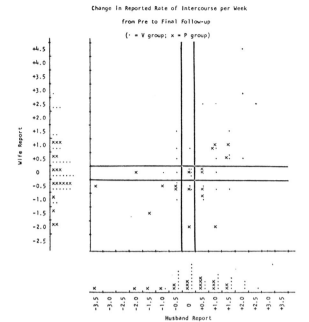

FIGURE 3

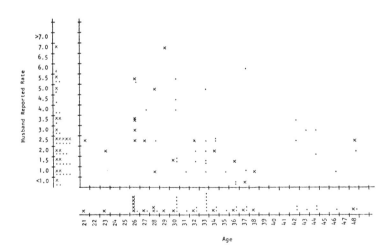

FIGURE 4

37

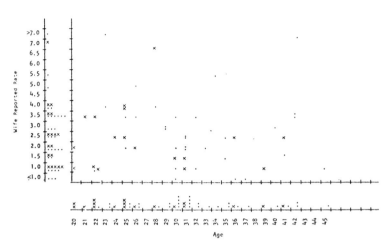

Age of Wife vs. Reported Rate of Intercourse per Week

(· = V group; x = P group)

FIGURE 5

preferred). Table 5 indicates the distribution of subjects in the two groups, by percentages, according to their degree of satisfaction with rate. Possibly because of the relatively small sample sizes, there is no statistically significant change (Chi square) in number of satisfied husbands or wives from initial interview to final interview. The P group shows a tendency toward increased satisfaction, and the V group shows a tendency toward decreased satisfaction. Especially noteworthy is the marked increase in number of sated wives of unsatisfied husbands in the V group, a trend that is not found in the P group. A somewhat more optimistic impression of change in sexual satisfaction was obtained from direct clinical assessment. Following systematic review of all available data, each couple was rated clinically (by two raters) as to whether they showed improvement, negligible change, or deterioration in overall sexual adjustment (Table 6). In general, both groups showed more improvement than deterioration, and the V group showed more change, both positive and negative, than the P group.

During the final interview, the women were asked to estimate the percentage of time they were experiencing orgasm with intercourse. Their responses are summarized in Table 7. Forty-eight per cent of

TABLE 3

Product Moment Correlations between Indicated Variables

Variable	Rate of intercourse as stated by			
	Husband		Wife	
	Initial interview	Final interview	Initial interview	Final interview
V group				
Age of husband...................	−.30	−.22	−.28	−.23
Age of wife......................	−.43*	−.34	−.46*	−.32
Years married...................	−.31	−.10	−.21	−.09
P group				
Age of husband...................	−.31	−.32	−.30	−.12
Age of wife......................	−.24	−.26	−.16	−.04
Years married...................	−.35	−.23	−.14	−.05

* indicates $p < .05$.

TABLE 4

Parameters of Sexual Intercourse

	Median	Low Extreme	High Extreme	Mean	S.D.
Frequency of intercourse, per week					
V husbands, initial interview	1.5	0.25	4.5	1.96	1.20
P husbands, initial interview	2.5	1.5	5.5	2.81	1.10
V wives, initial interview	1.75	0.25	4.5	2.08	1.33
P wives, initial interview	2.5	1.5	6.0	2.72	1.15
V husbands, final interview	2.5	0.25	6.0	2.52	1.56
P husbands, final interview	2.5	0.5	7.0	2.76	1.60
V wives, final interview	2.5	0.25	9.0	2.69	1.76
P wives, final interview	2.25	1.0	7.0	2.43	1.44
Duration of intercourse, minutes					
V husbands, final interview	22.5	5.0	60.0	23.7	12.5
P husbands, final interview	25.0	10.0	60.0	24.7	11.1
V wives, final interview	20.0	5.0	120.0	26.5	22.0
P wives, final interview	30.0	10.0	52.5	26.6	10.2
Penetration to ejaculation, minutes					
V husbands, final interview	5.0	1.0	12.5	5.7	3.73
P husbands, final interview	3.5	1.0	12.5	5.2	3.91
V wives, final interview	4.0	0.75	15.0	5.0	3.76
P wives, final interview	3.75	0.3	17.5	5.3	4.77

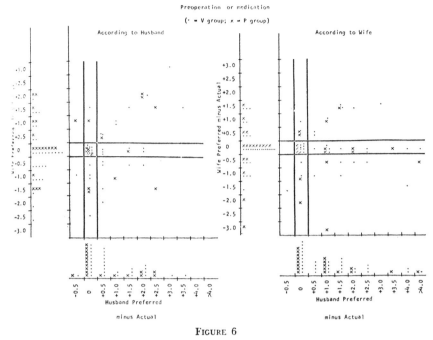

Difference between Preferred and Reported Rates of Intercourse per Week

Preoperation or medication

(· = V group; x = P group)

FIGURE 6

the P wives and 37 per cent of the V wives reported some incidence of multiple orgasm. While this was most common in the high-responsive women (those responding to intercourse with orgasm a high percentage of the time), it was also reported by some women whose responsiveness to intercourse was normally low. The subjects were also questioned concerning the different methods of stimulation that had led to orgasm at any time in their lives (Table 8) and the kinds of fantasies that accompanied intercourse and masturbation. The reported use of orgastic techniques other than intercourse, before and after change of contraceptive method, are summarized in Table 10. Problems of frigidity of the wife or impotence of the husband are summarized in Table 11.

The number of subjects admitting to extramarital relationships are tabulated in Table 12, according to whether such relationships occurred exclusively before use of the present contraceptive method, exclusively after, or both. Reasons given for not having extramarital affairs are shown in Table 13. Fear of pregnancy is not listed as a

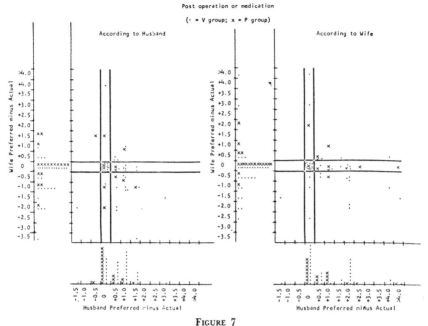

Difference between Preferred and Reported Rates of Intercourse per Week

Post operation or medication

(· = V group; x = P group)

FIGURE 7

TABLE 5

Per Cent of Couples Reporting Indicated Degrees of Correspondence between Preferred and Actual Frequency of Intercourse at Initial Interview (Pre) and at Final Interview (Post)

Wife	Husband						Total	
	Unsatisfied		Satisfied		Sated			
	P	V	P	V	P	V	P	V
Sated								
Pre	17	10	17	6	0	0	33	16
Post	11	39	0	6	0	0	11	45
Satisfied								
Pre	22	26	22	23	0	3	44	52
Post	22	32	39	10	6	0	67	42
Unsatisfied								
Pre	0	26	17	6	6	0	22	32
Post	0	3	22	6	0	3	22	13
Total								
Pre	39	61	56	36	6	3	100	100
Post	33	74	61	23	6	3	100	100

41

TABLE 6

Per Cent of Subjects with Indicated Changes in Clinically Rated
Overall Sexual Adjustment

Direction of Change	Group	
	P	V
Improved............................	39	61
No Change...........................	52	17
Deteriorated.........................	9	22

TABLE 7

Per Cent of Women Reporting Indicated Frequency of Orgasm during Intercourse,
at Time of Final Interview

Frequency of Orgasm	V Group	P Group
75–100%	54	65
50–75%	20	17
<50%	15	13
Never	12	4

separate category in Table 13, since it was cited by only one man and one woman in the entire study sample.

DISCUSSION

Agreement between Husband and Wife Reports

Since husband and wife were often describing, independently, the same behavioral events, comparisons of their answers should provide some evidence about the reliability of the information obtained (Winokur and Gaston, 1961). The correlations in Table 2 indicate that there is high agreement between husband and wife concerning frequency of intercourse, but there is less consistency of agreement on other parameters of the sexual relationship. With regard to preferred rate of intercourse, either the effectiveness of contraception or the participation in the research study (with its tendency to focus the couple's attention on their sexual relationship) tended to increase each respondent's awareness of the spouse's preferred rate. Interestingly, the greatest change in the V group concerned wife's awareness of the husband's preferences, while the P group husbands became more sensitized to the wife's preferences (Table 2). Another marked group difference concerned data on duration of intercourse from

TABLE 8

Per Cent of Women Responding with Orgasm to Indicated Stimulation
at Some Time in Life

(Responses exclusively to only one type of stimulation are shown in parentheses)

Type of Stimulation	V Wives	P Wives
Intercourse	90	91
(Intercourse only)	(7)	(9)
Manual stimulation by partner	76	87
Masturbation	32	48
(Masturbation only)	(2)	(0)
Oral-genital stimulation by partner	27	48
Dreams	29	39
(Dreams only)	(2)	(0)
Other	5	4
No experience of orgasm	2	4

TABLE 9

Per Cent of Subjects Reporting Indicated Primary Content of Fantasies during
Intercourse and during Masturbation

Primary Object of Fantasies	During Intercourse				During Masturbaion			
	V		P		V		P	
	♂	♀	♂	♀	♂	♀	♂	♀
Spouse as sexual partner	7	7	4	4	2	0	4	0
Spouse or other (unspecified) as sexual partner	5	0	9	9	20	7	48	9
Sexual partner other than spouse	10	2	9	0	7	5	17	9
Person(s) of opposite sex, but not necessarily as sexual partner	12	7	13	0	24	7	17	0
Self or own sensations	0	5	0	4	2	0	0	0
Stories, dreams, pictures	0	2	0	4	10	2	0	4
Non-sexual content or objects	5	2	0	13	0	0	0	0
No fantasies admitted	61	73	65	65	34	78*	13	78**

* 66 per cent did not admit to use of masturbation at any time in life.

** 52 per cent did not admit to use of masturbation at any time in life.

penetration to ejaculation and on total duration of intercourse, defined as "including foreplay and afterplay." The P group showed little agreement about total duration, but high agreement about length of pre-ejaculatory intromission. Exactly the opposite result was obtained in the V group, with high agreement about total length of intercourse but virtually no agreement about period of intromission (Table 2). The reasons for these differences are not apparent to us.

TABLE 10

Per Cent of Couples Reporting Use of Orgastic Techniques other than Intercourse

Technique	Before Change of Contraception		After Change of Contraception	
	P Group	V Group	P Group	V Group
Manual stimulation of husband	65	59	83	59
Manual stimulation of wife	61	61	74	61
Oral-genital stimulation of husband	48	46	65	54
Oral-genital stimulation of wife	52	51	65	44
Anal intercourse	17	10	13	15
Masturbation, husband	52	32	39	29
Masturbation, wife	9	10	9	12

TABLE 11

Number of Subjects Reporting Problems with Frigidity or with Impotence

Group	No. of Couples	Occasional Impotence		Frigidity			
				Pre		Post	
		Pre	Post	Complete	Inter-mittent	Complete	Inter-mittent
V	41	3	7	3	15	5	10
P	23	0	1	1	7	1	7

TABLE 12

Number of Subjects Reporting Extramarital Affairs

	♂		♀	
	V	P	V	P
No extramarital relations admitted	28	13	36	20
Affairs prior to but not during study	10	7	5	3
Affairs prior to and during study	3	0	0	0
Affairs only after beginning of study	0	3	0	0
Total	41	23	41	23

Retrospective subjective estimates of sexual parameters would thus appear to be imprecise at best. Reducing to a single average figure the frequency of sexual relations as they occur in a typical somewhat chaotic household of young children, periodic menstruation, aperiodic illness, business and social distractions, etc., is a somewhat nebulous task. Similarly, duration of intromission to time of ejacula-

TABLE 13
Per Cent of Subjects Indicated Reasons for Marital Fidelity

Reason	No Extramarital Experimence				Extramarital Experience			
	♂		♀		♂		♀	
	V	P	V	P	V	P	V	P
Fear of disrupting effect on family--marital relationship and children	43	46	31	35	31	30	60	33
Moral objections	46	23	43	45	8	40	40	33
Affection for present spouse	29	31	58	40	0	20	0	33
Adequate satisfaction with present spouse	50	23	17	25	8	10	0	0
No interest in, desire for, or "need for" other partners	14	31	44	45	23	10	20	33
Practical considerations								
Insufficient opportunity or time	18	15	3	5	15	30	20	0
Insufficient money	4	8	0	0	8	0	0	0
Miscellaneous								
Fear of general discovery	7	8	0	5	8	0	0	0
No desire to repeat previous experience	0	0	0	0	0	10	20	33
Fear of disease or pregnancy or impotence	7	8	0	5	8	0	0	0
No "gumption"	4	0	0	0	0	0	0	0
Desire to avoid involvement	4	0	0	0	0	0	0	0

tion and total duration of intercourse vary considerably in time from one experience to another and occur during an interval when atten tion is not likely to be critically focused on time estimation. In all these respects, it is apparent that the nature of the data to be reduced to single average figures is such as to introduce much ambiguity and some inevitable unreliability. When these contingencies are con sidered, the moderately high correlations in Table 2 and consistencies in averages in Table 4 suggest that the data obtained in the present tandem method of interviewing husband and wife provided at least some approximation of an accurate account of the sexual activity of these couples.

Factors Affecting Frequency of Intercourse

When effect of age on frequency of intercourse was examined (Table 3 and Figures 4 and 5), the expected negative relationship (Kinsey, et al., 1948) was consistently found. The correlations with age were relatively low, however, and reached statistical significance only in the comparison of age of V group wives to reported rate of intercourse prior to husband's vasectomy. From Table 3, it can be seen that effective non-coital contraception tended to reduce the correlations between age and frequency, especially in the V group. A possible explanation for this trend would be that in a population using coital and somewhat unreliable methods of contraception, increasing concern about pregnancy with age could contribute to a decreasing rate of intercourse, a contribution that would be removed by the effective non-coital methods of the present study.

By approximately four months after initiation of effective, non-coital contraception, both groups showed an average increase in frequency of intercourse (Figure 4). By final follow-up, however, much of this gain had been lost (Figure 5), especially for the P group, who then showed essentially no change from initial rates (Table 4). The V group maintained some positive gain in rate, sufficient to elevate mean frequency from an initial figure significantly below the P group, to an essentially equal rate at final follow-up (Table 4). While also distinctly dissatisfied with previous methods of contraception (Rodgers, et al., July 1965), the P group would seem to have been less inhibited in their rate of sexual intercourse prior to initiation of the present study than was the V group. From these data we infer that effective contraception can result in more frequent sexual experiences in couples who are markedly inhibited because of concern about pregnancy. Nevertheless, elimination of fear of pregnancy does not result in dramatic increase in frequency of coitus (Figure 5 and Table 4).

The complexity of the relationship between sexual satisfaction, contraception, and rate of intercourse is indicated by the data in Table 5. Preoperatively, 61 per cent of the V group men preferred a higher rate of intercourse than they were experiencing. Postoperatively, when fear of pregnancy was no longer a factor and when in fact rate of intercourse had increased (Table 4), the percentage of unsatisfied V group husbands had risen to 74 per cent. Their dissatisfaction possibly reflects counteractive concerns about masculinity (Ziegler, et al., 1966). At the same time, the number of sated wives of this same group rose from 16 to 45 per cent. Overall, discrepancy between preferred and actual rate of intercourse increased for the V group, couples for whom the mechanics of contraception were most completely divorced from the coital act. The P group provides evidence that non-coital contraception does not inevitably result in dis-

46

satisfaction with rate of intercourse, however. Initially, one-third of the P group wives reported a higher frequency of intercourse than they desired (Table 5). After the wives began using the pills, which might theoretically have made them more vulnerable to their husbands' excessive demands, the frequency of sated wives dropped to 11 per cent. During the same interim, the number of unsatisfied P group husbands declined slightly. Overall, there was an increase in numbers of satisfied husbands and satisfied wives in the P group, even though frequency of intercourse did not change (Tables 4 and 5).

Further complicating the question of the nature of change in sexual activity and satisfaction from beginning to end of the study are the results of the clinical ratings of sexual adjustment (Table 6). These ratings reveal a generally greater frequency of improvement than deterioration, although some negative changes occur. The V group apparently experienced the strongest reaction to the change in procedure, some responding favorably and some unfavorably, with fewer than one-fifth showing essentially no change in adjustment. In contrast, over half of the P group showed essentially no change. The present data do not indicate whether the greater reaction of the V group was a consequence of pre-existing differences from the P group. or of differences between the operation and the pills as contraceptive procedures, although this complicated question has been considered in a previous report (Ziegler, et al., 1966). The rather inconsistent and somewhat contradictory results from the two groups suggest that sweeping generalizations cannot accurately be made about the relationships between coitus and likelihood of conception and between sexual satisfaction and sexual behavior.

Orgastic Responsiveness and Orgastic Techniques

The data in Tables 7 through 10 are essentially normative and require little interpretation. Four of the 64 women had not experienced climax during intercourse. Two women reported the occurrence of spontaneous orgasms (one during spastic colitis episodes), and one woman reported experiencing climax while delivering a baby. Although the differences are not statistically significant, there is a trend in all of the tables suggesting that the P group wives are somewhat more responsive and somewhat more experienced with a variety of orgastic techniques than are the V group wives. Most women (87 per cent of the V group and 87 per cent of the P group) had experienced orgasm from more than one type of stimulation. Forty-three per cent of the P group wives and 24 per cent of the V group wives reported ability to respond with orgasm to coital, manual, and oral stimulatory techniques. Although personal reactions, relationships with partners, and other physical sensations associated with the particular type of stimulation contributed to the ultimate subjective response, the essential characteristics of the orgasm or climax per se were generally reported to be similar for the various stimulatory techniques employed. Several women volunteered that they had been confused by medical references suggesting that clitoral and vaginal orgasms differ from each other, a difference that they had failed to experience. These clinical data would thus seem to lend some support to the considerable physiological data by Masters and Johnson (1966) concerning the nature of female erotic arousal and climax.

At least occasional use of non-coital techniques of stimulation to orgasm was reported by a large proportion of the subjects (Table 10). Thirty per cent of subjects admitting use of such techniques prior to change of contraceptive method reported doing so because of fear that pregnancy might result from coitus. The proportion of subjects admitting use was approximately the same in each group and for each sex. The failure of effective contraception to reduce reported incidence of such non-coital techniques (Table 10), however, suggests that stated fear of pregnancy was, at least in part, a rationalization for pleasurable but somewhat taboo behavior. Reports of such behavior in fact tended to increase following the shift to non-coital methods of contraception. The subjects may, of course, have been more cooperative in revealing relevant data on the follow-up interview, and the initial interviews might have tended to stimulate curiosity concerning other methods of arousal and to reduce inhibitions about trying other methods (as was alleged, supposedly jokingly, by two couples who had experimented with anal intercourse during the interval between interviews). But in any event, the data strongly suggest that fear of pregnancy is seldom the primary reason that couples use non-coital techniques of stimulation to orgasm, even when it is so rationalized.

Sixty-six per cent of all subjects denied the use of fantasies, daydreams, mental pictures, or other mental content during intercourse, and the proportions of subjects denying such activity were approximately the same for both groups and both sexes (Table 9). It was, however, the interviewer's impression that this was the most sensitive and guarded area in the sexual histories obtained. The fantasies that were reported by the husbands usually involved sexual intercourse and/or sexual play with a woman other than wife. One man stated that he had fantasies of wishing he could fly. Non-sexual content, such as arithmetic computations, was occasionally reported, and was described as a way of reducing excitement and prolonging the duration of intercourse. The women reported somewhat less specific fantasies than the men, although these also often involved erotic behavior with men other than husband. Other fantasies concerned "nasty girls dancing to excite men;" simply the satisfaction of being a woman; consideration of how well own performance compared to that of other women; contemplation of the futility of fighting about things in marriage; thoughts of being angry at husband; and imagery of chandeliers, castles, log cabins, and "fine wood pieces."

Fantasying during masturbation was acknowledged by 87 and 66 per cent of the P and the V group men, respectively, and by 74 and 88 per cent, respectively, of the P and V group women who reported use of masturbation. Own spouse was more often fantasied during masturbation than during intercourse, although thoughts of both men and women were typically of partner other than spouse. Several men and women reported thinking about erotic material they had read. One woman reported that she was stimulated "just by the idea of sexual intercourse."

Impotence and Frigidity

The data in Table 11 suggest that perhaps an occasional man may respond to certainty of contraception (or perhaps to vasectomy per se) with increased intermittent impotence. While one of the V group husbands who had reported previous intermittent problems with impotence indicated no recurrence of the problem after the operation, the other two reported no change, and five additional men reported some occurrences of impotence postoperative in the absence of similar problems preoperatively. In addition, one P group husband reported impotence problems at follow-up that had not been present initially, although he attributed this "to prostate trouble," and did not relate it to the contraceptive procedure of his wife. These reliable, non-coital contraceptive procedures apparently had little effect on the frigidity problems of the women. The subjects were deliberately allowed to define for themselves what was meant by frigidity, so that subjective distress or concern about wife's responsiveness would be the primary criterion. While it was closely related to orgastic responsiveness (Table 6), a few frequently responsive subjects complained of intermittent frigidity and some infrequently orgastic subjects did not. None of the P group wives reported either an increase in or an elimination of pre-existing frigidity problems, although four of the seven with mild problems reported some improvement after use of the pills. Effects were more varied in the V group wives. None without pre-existing problems of frigidity reported such problems postoperatively; three with such past history reported absence of problems postoperatively; and four others reported improvement, even though some problems remained. However, three of the V group wives reported increased frigidity problems postoperatively, including two who shifted from intermittent to complete frigidity. It should be recalled that an appreciable number of original study couples beginning use of pills were not included in the present report because they had discontinued use of the pills before the final follow-up interview. This group included some women whose responsiveness had not improved or had deteriorated post-medication. The present data do not warrant the interpretation, therefore, that use of pills leads on balance to increased responsiveness of the women. Conversely, even when the noncontinuous group is included, there is no evidence of an average trend toward marked deterioration of responsiveness.

Extramarital Affairs

The question of whether or not certainty of contraception leads to increased infidelity is of considerable cultural interest. Fear of extramarital impregnation has been assumed by some to inhibit extramarital sexual activity. Table 12 suggests that there is no marked increase in such affairs over the one to two year interval of effective contraception covered by the present study. Indeed, only two subjects list concern about pregnancy as a factor in their own marital fidelity (Table 13). Thirteen V group men, or 32 per cent of the total, admitted extramarital affairs. Of these, only three reported having had affairs postoperatively; and none of these three was inexperienced in such affairs preoperatively. Three, or 13 per cent, of the P group women admitted to previous experience with extramarital affairs; but none admitted any such experience since beginning the pills. Thus, in no reported case did effective contraception result in infidelity on the part of the protected person.

Five, or 12 per cent, of the V group women admitted past extramarital experiences and none admitted experiences after husband had had a vasectomy. Only with the husbands in the P group did extramarital affairs originate during the course of the study. All together, 10 (or 43 per cent) of the P group men reported extramarital sexual experiences and three of these (or 13 per cent) had their initial affairs after their wives began use of the pills. The number of men included is, of course, too low to permit any conclusions from this information. The data cannot rule out the possibility that some husbands may find their wives somewhat less attractive if they are known to be infertile. An equally plausible alternative explanation of the extramarital activities of the P group men would be that husbands of wives on pills are sensitized to the possible safe availability of other women who are also taking pills.

At the time of the follow-up interview, each respondent was asked either to give his or her reasons for remaining faithful to spouse or, if extramarital sexual experience had been reported, to give reasons why he or she had not used extramarital outlets more extensively. The responses are listed in Table 13. As is reflected in the table, many people gave more than one reason. The major categories offered were concerns about jeopardizing the integrity of the family, general standards of morality, affection for present spouse, and no interest in other possible partners. Only two subjects who had previously experienced extramarital liaisons gave adequate satisfaction with present spouse as a reason for fidelity, although this was a common reason given by the remaining subjects. Many more female than male respondents alleged no interest in other possible partners, perhaps suggesting more sated wives than husbands, but also possibly reflecting the reporting characteristics of female respondents. A number of respondents, more male than female, simply listed practical reasons, such as lack of opportunity, lack of time, lack of financial resources to fund extramarital activities, and difficulty in being able to manage having the right partner at the right place at the right time. One man feared that once he started extramarital sex experience, he would not be able to control himself. One feared it would lead to impotence, one feared it would lead to entangling emotional relationships, and several reported that extramarital experiences in the past had been upsetting and disruptive. One man complained that he had too little "gumption" to manage extramarital liaisons.

Overall, the conclusion seems reasonable that the subjects in the study sample as a whole were relatively willing to reveal extramarital affairs and that effective contraception did not lead to a dramatic increase in the incidence of such affairs. The present data suggest that fear of impregnation is a relatively minor factor in nonmarital sexual relationships and that cultural mores, practical considerations, and personal moral values concerning monogamy are of far more fundamental influence (Table 13). Whether or not long term experience with effective contraception would lead to increased exploration of extramarital liaisons cannot of course be ascertained from the present data.

SUMMARY

Actuarial information is reported concerning sexual experience, practices, and preferences of 41 men and their wives, interviewed shortly before the men had vasectomy operations for contraception (V group subjects), and 23 women and their husbands, interviewed shortly before the women initiated use of ovulation suppressors (P group subjects). Information from the same 128 respondents, obtained 12–24 months after continuous use of the new contraceptive precedure, is also reported and is assessed for evidence of effects of the shift to an effective, non-coital method of contraception. Respondents were predominantly middle and upper-middle class, young to middle-aged, white Americans, who seemed generally interested and cooperative in the study even though they had not anticipated the extent of interrogation about sexual matters. Interviewing of husband and wife was sequential, by the same interviewer, without opportunity for the couple to exchange information between interviews. Comparison of information obtained indicated a generally acceptable level of consistency of reporting.

Average rate of intercourse of the P group was essentially the same at final interviews as initially, suggesting that the change in contraceptive procedure had no enduring effect on frequency. Frequency of the V group, significantly below that of the P group initially, had risen to comparable levels by final follow-up, suggesting that effective non-coital contraception can elevate a previously depressed rate. Effective non-coital contraception tended to reduce the expected negative correlation between age of respondent and frequency of intercourse. When satisfaction with frequency of intercourse was determined by comparing stated preferred rate with reported actual rate, the P group showed an increase in number of both satisfied husbands and satisfied wives, even though mean frequency of intercourse did not change. In contrast, by final follow-up more V group husbands considered that they were not having intercourse often enough and more V group wives considered that they were having intercourse too often. Both initially and at final interview, most couples reported at least occasional use of non-coital orgastic techniques. While occasionally rationalized as due to fear of pregnancy initially, these non-coital techniques were reported at least as often after vasectomy or use of ovulation suppressors as before, suggesting that intrinsic interest rather than fear of pregnancy was a primary determining factor. About 85 per cent of the women in the study reported ability to respond with orgasm to both intercourse and some other stimulatory technique. Four more of the V group men and one more of the P group men reported at least occasional impotence at the final interview than had noted this problem initially. The possibility therefore cannot be ruled out that either the vasectomy operation per se or effective contraception per se contributed to the increasing incidence of impotence, although the number of respondents involved is too low to warrant drawing even tentative conclusions. Essentially the same number of women reported intermittent or self-defined frigidity problems at follow-up as had reported such problems in the initial interview, suggesting that the change in contraceptive procedure had little effect on frigidity problems. Approximately 10 per cent of the female respondents reported complete frigidity, defined as inability to have orgasm during intercourse. Certainty of contraception did not stimulate a reportable increase in extramarital sexual activity, since none of the women on pills and none of the men with vasectomy operations without prior extramarital experience sought such contacts after they had become infertile. Three V group men, however, continued extramarital affairs that had been initiated preoperatively, and three of the P group husbands had initial affairs after their wives began use of the pills (an incidence that may not be beyond expectation in a group of 23 couples over a two-year period). While few generalizations are possible from the study, the conclusion seems reasonable that effective contraception removed fear of pregnancy as both an inhibiting and a bargaining influence in the marriages, did not solve frigidity problems, did not lead to a reduction in variety of orgastic techniques employed, and did not stimulate increased extramarital activity. It thus would seem not to solve as many problems as some might hope nor to create as many as others might fear.

References

KINSEY, A. C., POMEROY, W. B., AND MARTIN, C. E. *Sexual Behavior in the Human Male*. Philadelphia: W. B. Saunders, 1948.

LEHFELDT, H. Willful exposure to unwanted pregnancy. *American Journal of Obstetrics and Gynecology*, 1959, *78*: 661–5.

MASTERS, W. H. AND JOHNSON, VIRGINIA E. *Human Sexual Response*. Boston: Little, Brown, Co., 1966.

POLGAR, S. AND GUTTMACHER, A. F. A new chapter in family planning. *Columbia University Forum*, Fall 1966, 34–7.

RODGERS, D. A., ZIEGLER, F. J., ROHR, PATRICIA, AND PRENTISS, R. J. Sociopsychological characteristics of patients obtaining vasectomies from urologists. *Marriage and Family Living*, 1963, *25*: 331–5.

RODGERS, D. A., ZIEGLER, F. J., ALTROCCHI, J., AND LEVY, N. A longitudinal study of the psychosocial effects of vasectomy. *Marriage and the Family*, Feb. 1965, *27*: 59–64.

RODGERS, D. A., ZIEGLER, F. J., PRENTISS, R. J., AND MARTIN, P. L. Comparisons of nine contraceptive procedures by couples changing to vasectomy or ovulation suppression medication. *Journal of Sex Research*, July 1965, *1*: 87–96.

TIETZE, C. The clinical effectiveness of contraception. Third International Conference on Planned Parenthood, Report of the Proceedings, Bombay, India, 1952, 24–29.

TIETZE, C. The use-effectiveness of contraceptive methods. In: *Research in Family Planning*. C. V. Kiser (Ed.). Princeton: Princeton University Press, 1962.

WINOKUR, G. AND GASTON, W. R. Sex, anger and anxiety: Intrapersonal interaction in married couples. *Diseases of the Nervous System*, 1961, *22*: 1–5.

ZIEGLER, F. J., RODGERS, D. A., AND KRIEGSMAN, SALI ANN. Effect of vasectomy on psychological functioning. *Psychosomatic Medicine*, 1966, *28*: 50–63.

SEMEN EXAMINATIONS
AFTER VASECTOMY

J. C. SMITH

The letter from Mr. Temple and Mr. Jameson (Dec. 12, p. 1258) reporting spermatozoa (of unstated numbers) in the third semen specimen after vasectomy following two azoospermic specimens is likely to cause a lot of worry to vasectomists and their patients. It is highly probable that the worry is unnecessary, since the finding of a few non-motile spermatozoa in the semen after vasectomy does not imply fertility.

The length to which one should go to prove infertility after vasectomy is debatable, and statistically it seems probable that an occasional patient will produce an occasional sperm after even five or six negative specimens. Recanalisation of the vas is a separate problem, but if carried to its logical conclusion this argument would lead to regular semen examination indefinitely—totally defeating the object of the operation, which is to free the patient from worry.

Two azoospermic specimens following vasectomy give virtual certainty that the patient is sterile, and the addition of one further negative specimen adds little to this confidence. Vasectomists must face the fact that, even taking every possible precaution, recanalisation will occur in very exceptional cases, but that placing undue emphasis on this possibility to the patient may well defeat the object of the operation.

VOLUNTARY STERILISATION

John M. Beazley   W. J. Fraser

INTRODUCTION

UNTIL recently, any woman seeking sterilisation at the university unit of this hospital made her request at the gynæcological outpatients department, or, more commonly, while attending the antenatal clinic. When sterilisation seemed advisable her name was added to the surgical waiting-list. Commonly, tubal occlusion was done during the early puerperium. Before surgery, the husband was given a brief explanation of the proposed operation, and obliged to sign a form consenting to the procedure. Otherwise, little attention was paid to the husband.

In June, 1967, consideration of the increasing number of requests for sterilisation, the increasing use of vasectomy in other centres, and the ignorance of many patients about family planning, led us to conclude that we should interview more husbands of women requesting sterilisation. We set up a special clinic for this purpose.

METHOD

All men or women requesting sterilisation were interviewed, together with their spouse. Each couple was seen twice.

At the first interview patients were invited to state what help they wanted. They were instructed briefly about contraceptive methods and the operations for vas ligation, and occlusion of the fallopian tubes.

At the second interview, the couple were invited to submit a precise request, either for contraception, or for vasectomy or tubal occlusion, and to provide reasons in support of their choice.

Each couple was questioned about age, nationality, religion, previous medical, surgical, gynæcological, and obstetric history, income, expenditure, social background, and contraceptive practices.

During the ensuing discussion, points raised for their consideration included: the permanence of an operation; the possibility of subsequent remorse, promiscuity, or disaffection arising between the partners; the possible death of one partner or of an existing or unborn child; possible dissatisfaction at the loss of any possible risk of pregnancy; divorce; possible alterations in religious practice.

Only after the second interview, when each couple had submitted their formal request, did we consider whether it seemed reasonable, and whether help could be offered for medical indications.

Between June, 1967, and October, 1968, we interviewed 96 couples. Most of them lived in a poor section of the community, which is served by this hospital. In 40% of the couples, one or both partners seemed to us to have less-than-average intelligence.

Contraceptive Practice

Only 15 of the couples interviewed had made any serious attempt to use effective contraception. Of the remainder, none had sought contraceptive advice

TABLE I—CONTRACEPTIVE PRACTICE

Contraception used				No. of couples
Frequently	..	..	..	..	15 *(15·6%)*
Very irregularly ..		..	..	..	29 *(30·2%)*
Never	..	..	..	..	52 *(54·2%)*
Total	..	..	..		96

TABLE II—REQUESTS FOR STERILISATION

Primary reason				No. of couples
Eugenic ..	..	..	..	..	3 *(3·1%)*
Therapeutic	..	..	..	..	17 *(17·7%)*
Familial ..	..	..	..	..	72 *(75%)*
Convenience	..	..	..	..	4 *(4·2%)*
Total	..	..	..		96

previously. A request for sterilisation was the help first sought by more than half the group (table I).

Requests for Sterilisation

Table II shows the primary indications for sterilisation grouped under the four headings proposed by the Simon Population Trust.[1]

Of 3 requests for eugenic reasons, 1 of the couples had had five children: three grossly abnormal, one phenotypically normal but abnormal genetically, and one normal. The father had a significant autosomal abnormality. Of the 2 remaining couples, 1 had had five children of whom three died with fibrocystic disease. The other had two living children, both of whom were born with congenital adrenal hyperplasia.

17 patients sterilised for medical indications included 3 couples with severe rhesus incompatibility, and 14 couples where the wife had an incapacitating illness (mitral stenosis, chronic pyelonephritis, respiratory insufficiency, severe epilepsy, or diabetes).

Age Incidence and Parity

76 couples requested sterilisation for familial reasons or for convenience.

In this series, the " age plus parity " index was

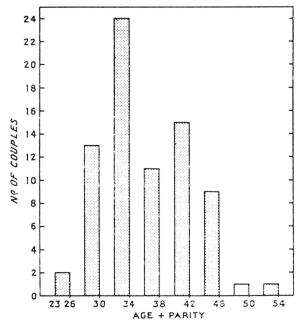

Distribution of age and parity index.
This index is calculated by adding the age of the wife to the total number of children.

under 35 in 39 requests, and in almost half of these the index was under 31 (see figure).

Most young patients with small families were persuaded to use contraception. 5 couples decided in favour of sterilisation despite their youth and small family, but only in 2 instances was sterilisation done.

Vasectomy

Vas ligation was done on 12 men, the predominant indication being " familial " (10 cases), " eugenic " and " convenience " being the indications in the other 2.

4 more husbands requesting vasectomy would have been operated on if the wife had not objected to the proposed surgery. 1 of these women, who had oligomenorrhœa, was so unsure about the efficacy of vasectomy that she claimed even if her husband was sterilised she would think she was pregnant every time menstruation was overdue. The remaining 3 women were so concerned about their husbands' psychological reactions to vasectomy, that tubal ligation was thought to be preferable for these couples.

Amongst the 96 couples requesting sterilisation there were 3 husbands who, within the preceding six months,

TABLE III—RESULTS OF INTERVIEW

Outcome	No. of couples
Wife sterilised	46 (47·9%)
Husband sterilised	12 (12·6%)
Referred for contraception	18 (18·7%)
Did not reattend	20 (20·8%)
Total	96

had undergone an inguinal hernia repair, at which operation the surgeon had purposely avoided ligating the vas.

We find very few Jamaican men are prepared to accept responsibility for birth control, and will rarely countenance the possibility of vasectomy.

Results of Interview

Table III summarises the results of interviewing 96 couples. 20 couples did not attend for a second interview: under the pre-vasectomy regimen J. M. B. would have advised tubal occlusion in 15 cases and contraception in 5.

DISCUSSION

To assess the true need for sterilisation and the most appropriate operative method, and to avoid undesirable postoperative sequelæ, couples requesting sterilisation should be interviewed together. We believe that unwillingness of either the husband or wife to attend for interview may be regarded, usually, as a contra-indication to sterilisation.

One advantage of a two-interview system is that couples can consider all the facts before coming to a final decision. In some difficult cases we found it helpful to defer a final decision until the youngest child was one year old. The couple were assisted with suitable contraception during the interim, and their case was reviewed at three-monthly intervals.

It is debatable whether a two-interview system always results in the best management. Among the 20 couples who did not return for their second interview, 15 women probably would have undergone tubal occlusion had they not been required to attend with their husbands or on two occasions.

It is often difficult to distinguish precisely between familial and therapeutic indications for sterilisation, especially when anxiety can adversely affect the mental or physical health of the husband and wife. Neither vas ligation nor tubal occlusion for purely familial reasons is permitted under the National Health Service.[1] It is our experience, however, that most tubal occlusions performed under the N.H.S. are in fact done mainly for familial reasons but justified, if necessary, by invoking rather vague therapeutic indications. Vasectomy for familial reasons rarely seems to be done under the N.H.S., although similar vague therapeutic indications could be invoked in most instances. In practice, we have found this difference in management sometimes influences couples to request tubal occlusion to avoid the significant financial burden of vasectomy done privately.

We believe that requests for sterilisation, especially for familial reasons, but also for convenience, will increase in the future. People now marry young and quickly have the desired number of children. Many parents subsequently rely on contraception to limit their family. Some intelligent, young couples would, however, prefer the freedom offered by sterilisation. Optimal family size, or the acceptability of a calculated genetic risk are further very personal matters, and, in our experience, they too may lead to a conflict of opinion which the clinician often finds difficult to resolve impersonally. More than 700 years ago St. Thomas Aquinas suggested families should restrict their children to a number they can nourish, protect, and educate until adulthood. We consider this to be good advice still.

Although vasectomy is more simple, safer, cheaper for the State, and quicker than tubal occlusion, it does not confer immediate protection,[2] and it is inappropriate if either the husband or wife believe the operation may change the man in some indefinable way. We would urge general surgeons, however, to inquire about the possibility of vasectomy before they operate on men with families to repair inguinal hernias, and also to discuss tubal occlusion with parous women who are to undergo laparotomy.

In this series, men, even professional men, often failed to distinguish between fertility and virility or impotence.[3] Thus, vasectomy, when mentioned at the first interview, was met by many husbands with expressions of incredulous disbelief, or else ignorance and male prejudice. They rarely objected to tubal occlusion on their wives. Most male patients, however, discovered in themselves genuine, if ill-defined antagonism to vas ligation.

In our view, many Englishmen are not yet wholly prepared to accept male sterilisation; nor should they be persuaded to accept vasectomy against their will.

REFERENCES

1. Blacker, C. P., Jackson, L. N. *Lancet*, 1966, i, 971.
2. Hanley, H. G. *ibid*. 1968, ii, 207.
3. Peberdy, M. *ibid*. 1968, i, 1363.

Vasectomy: Research Proposal

ANNE ROE

The letters by Nag and Shokeir (3 Apr.) agree with my belief that the combination of a vasectomy and preservation of semen presents the surest and easiest method of contraception without any of the problems caused by the side effects of hormonal substances, not to mention the numerous drawbacks of other techniques. I suggest that (as a free public service) any couple not desiring children at the moment be offered the opportunity of depositing the man's sperm in a sperm bank (its eventual use being limited to him alone), to be followed by his having a vasectomy.

There is another area of research which deserves full investigation and top priority; that is, to determine the length of time during which viable sperm continue to be produced after vasectomy and satisfactory techniques for their retrieval. If any man can continue to be his own sperm bank for a reasonable period of time, many difficulties associated with sperm preservation would be obviated. As a precaution, sperm should, of course, be preserved in advance of the vasectomy in the event a man's fertile period following the operation is relatively brief.

In either case when the time came that *both* partners wanted a child, insemination of the woman would be a simple matter, and it is obvious that the free consent of both would be necessary. The relaxation of abortion laws frees women from having to bear unwanted children; this system would free them from the pill or other methods, and from what is in practice usually their responsibility. It would also protect unwilling fathers, whose situation has been generally disregarded, and so prevent the birth of any child who is not really wanted by both parents at the time he is born. Such a system on a national scale would introduce no class or ethnic discrimination. The problems involved are not technical, but educational, administrative, and political. My conjecture is that the young generation would accept this solution once they understood that vasectomy does not interfere with normal intercourse.

ABORTION AND STERILIZATION
Status of the Law in Mid-1970

The battle against restrictive abortion laws now has a second front. In the past two years there have been several successful challenges—on grounds of constitutionality—to such laws in the courts.

The importance of this development is that it raises fundamental questions about the extent to which the state may interfere with individuals' decisions concerning their own bodies.

There is a crucial distinction between consideration of abortion law revision in the legislature and deliberations by a court in a prosecution for violation of the abortion law, when it is asserted by the defendant that the law conflicts with constitutionally protected rights. In the legislative forum the contending forces are seeking to garner majority support for legislative change or for maintenance of the *status quo.* Often an accommodation, somewhat acceptable to both sides, but fully satisfactory to neither, is reached through negotiation. In the judicial forum, when the constitutional challenge to the abortion law is

made, the court must consider the individual defendant's legal rights. These can take precedence over any law, even one that all legislators favored strongly.

People v. Belous,[1] dealt with the conviction of a physician who had been found guilty of violating the abortion law that was in effect in the state of California before 1967. The conviction was reversed on the ground that the statute violated due process because its language was vague and uncertain.

The defendant physician had directed a young couple to another physician for an abortion. He believed that otherwise the woman would have gone to Tijuana for an abortion. The defendant stated his belief that her life would have been in considerably greater danger from an abortion performed there than from one performed by the physician to whom he referred the couple.

The California statute then in effect authorized abortions by li-

[1] 80 California Reporter 354 (1969).

62

censed physicians only when "necessary to preserve" life. The California Supreme Court held that the words "necessary to preserve" did not create a proper standard and were not clearly definable. One of the basic concepts in the guarantee of due process of law is that there be a reasonable degree of certainty in law, in criminal law especially.

The lack of such certainty in the legislation places the physician in a dilemma. A physician decides an abortion for the woman is legally justified because he believes it is necessary to preserve her life. Subsequently, he is prosecuted for performing an illegal abortion—a felony —and convicted. He is then subject to criminal penalties and the loss of his right to practice. It has been asserted, then, that a physician would tend to decide close questions conservatively. Even though a patient's life might be at stake, he might decide against performing an abortion simply because of his important interest in preserving his professional standing. The risks of an erroneous decision not to provide an abortion, even though it was "necessary to preserve" the woman's life, did not include possible criminal sanction, although liability for malpractice could follow.

The court said that, with a person's life at stake, the delegation of decision-making power to an individual who was subject to pressure to select a course of conduct to minimize his potential criminal responsibility, violated the fourteenth amendment of the U.S. Constitution. The physician's direct personal involvement established a conflict of interest; the threat of prosecution could affect his professional judgment.

In an even more far-reaching case,[2] a federal district court held the abortion statute of the District of Columbia unconstitutional on the ground that it is an unwarranted infringement on the right of privacy of a licensed physician's woman patient. The judge drew largely on the recognition of the right of privacy in a decision by the U.S. Supreme Court in which the court held that a Connecticut statute forbidding the use of contraceptive devices was constitutionally inapplicable to married persons.[3] He reached the conclusion that the District of Columbia abortion law, which declares an abortion illegal unless it is necessary to preserve the life or health of the woman, interferes with both the woman's right of privacy and the right granted the physician by the issuance to him of a license under the medical practice act.

Challenges to other state abortion statutes are being made on other theories. One such case may soon reach the U.S. Supreme Court. If it does, it will present the basic issue of whether the state may make illegal the performance of an abortion by a licensed physician if the woman has capacity to make a decision and has given her consent.

No one can do more than guess about the number of illegal abor-

[2] United States v. Vuitch, 305 F. Supp. 1032 (1969).
[3] Griswold v. Connecticut, 381 U.S. 479 (1965).

63

tions, but there are few who believe that revised abortion laws have appreciably reduced the number of illegal abortions in the ten or more states that have broadened grounds for legal abortions. For this reason, and because of the relative success of recent court actions, legislation that eliminates completely the need to establish medical justification for abortion has been enacted in some states and is being seriously considered in several others.[4] These would declare legal all abortions performed by physicians on consenting women, at least until the fetus is likely to be viable. And even at such time, protection of the woman's life would still be grounds for abortion. It is likely that a ruling by the Supreme Court that a state may not declare criminal an abortion performed by a physician in conformity with the woman's desires would have the effect of nullifying both the newer laws, with expanded grounds for medical justification, and the older, more restrictive ones.

The law on voluntary sterilization, often referred to as sterilization of convenience, has also been undergoing change. Two of the three states that until recently had laws declaring sterilization of convenience illegal have repealed them,[5] and only in Utah are such procedures now declared illegal.

There had been concern in states without laws on the subject that voluntary sterilization was contrary to public policy. In a number of opinions of state attorneys-general and in several state court decisions, there have been statements declaring such procedures to be not inconsistent with public policy. Furthermore, several states have enacted legislation specifically authorizing sterilizations of convenience, performed by physicians in hospitals after appropriate consent has been obtained.[6]

The substantial changes in the law relating to abortion and sterilization of convenience reflect the changes in the views of the public about such procedures. These are based on wider acceptance of concepts of individual rights in areas that are asserted to be private and beyond the jurisdiction of government. Perhaps the extent of the shift in attitudes is best exemplified by a recent suit in California in which a medically indigent couple asserted that they were entitled to have a sterilization of convenience provided by the public health and welfare authorities.

The couple asserted that they had as many children already as they could properly care for and that they were unable to secure the sterilization only because they lacked the financial resources to employ a private physician. They pointed out that persons who were financially able could obtain such services through private medical practitioners. Part of the argument was buttressed on the concepts of due process and equal protection guaranteed by the constitutions of

---

[4] E.g. Act 1, Hawaii Laws 1970; Chap. 127, New York Laws 1970.
[5] Connecticut and Kansas.

[6] E.g. N.C. Gen. Stat., 90-271 et. seq.

64

the state of California and the United States.

The California appellate court declined to rule on the question of whether the public authorities were obliged to provide a sterilization at public expense to medically indigent persons, but only because it found that the record before the lower court on the question was insufficient, and that the issue had not been adequately explored in the prior proceeding.[7] The court did not dismiss the argument out of hand.

Predictions about developing law involve risks, as do all predictions. However, it may well be that in a few years, not only sterilizations of convenience but also, non-therapeutic abortions, as well, will be freely available, at public expense, to those who lack financial resources to pay for them.

[7] Jessin v. County of Shasta, 70 California Reporter 359 (1969).

65

A Male Sterilization Clinic

PAULINE JACKSON, M.B., B.S., D.C.H.

BETSON PHILLIPS, M.B., B.CH., B.SC.

ELIZABETH PROSSER, M.B., B.S., D.R.C.O.G.

H. O. JONES, M.S., F.R.C.S.

V. R. TINDALL, F.R.C.S., M.R.C.O.G.

D. L. CROSBY, F.R.C.S.

I. D. COOKE, M.R.C.O.G.

J. M. McGARRY, M.R.C.O.G.

R. W. REES, F.R.C.S.

Introduction

Until recently the practicality of male sterilization has been clouded in the medical mind by its possible but never proved illegality, and in the lay mind by its association with castration. In 1960, however, the medical defence societies were advised that male sterilization was not unlawful, and soon afterwards the Simon Population Trust launched a successful campaign to promote awareness of vasectomy. In April of this year the Secretary of State for Health and Social Security announced that vasectomy could be carried out under the National Health Service if the health of the husband or wife was in danger.

The need for fertility control in Britain passed rapidly from private to public recognition in the 1960s, culminating in the **Family Planning Act of 1967**. The desire for permanent family limitation seems to be spreading, and female sterilization is increasingly requested and practised. The interest in male sterilization is shown in the Chart. Those put on the waiting list were, with very few exceptions, couples who lived within a reasonable distance from Cardiff and who could return home on the evening the interview or operation took place.

Before the clinic was started the one surgeon undertaking vasectomy found that the demand was rapidly growing and also that assessing initially the couple's contraceptive needs was beyond his knowledge. He asked the Family Planning Association for advice and this resulted in the setting up of a male sterilization clinic.

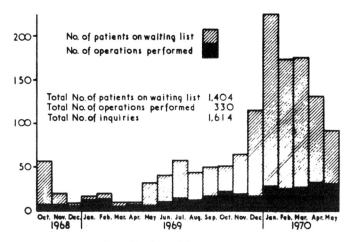

Trend in demand for vasectomy.

Many thousands of vasectomies have already been performed, but most of these have been carried out privately, and have therefore been beyond the financial means of most of the community. The Family Planning Association, which is a charitable and self-supporting organization, charged a fee of 15 guineas for the operation, but this was remitted or deferred whenever necessary. Of the 330 cases reported here no charge was made in 10%, and the fee was reduced in a further 9%. The aims of the clinic were to provide an additional method of contraception which was within the means of all, and also material for teaching and research.

Method

Selection

The doctor interviewing the couple had had training in contraception and psychosexual patterns. The discussion was designed to determine whether sterilization would promote the welfare of the whole family unit. A decision was made after many factors had been considered—medical, social, and emotional. The merits of both female and male sterilization were discussed, and close co-operation with the gynaecologists facilitated treatment for the wife, if thought necessary.

Each interview lasted 30 to 45 minutes. Information was recorded on the clinic form regarding the following questions.

Age of husband and wife
Years married
Past medical history:
    Husband—including hernia and genital abnormality
    Wife—general, obstetric

No. of children and ages
No. of abortions
No. of unplanned pregnancies

Previous contraception
- Oral
- Intrauterine device
- Diaphragm
- Sheath
- Coitus interruptus
- Other

Request for female sterilization
Couple's reason for permanent method
Coital frequency
Coital satisfaction { Husband / Wife
Coital difficulty { Husband / Wife
Consideration of death of child
Consideration of husband remarrying
Apparent relationship between husband and wife
Apparent attitude towards children
Comments by interviewer

Information Given to Couple

If vasectomy was agreed to, the couple were given information about the operation and its effects. They were told that it had to be regarded as irreversible, and a diagram helped to explain that sexual activity and desire remained unchanged. The importance of continuing to have intercourse to remove the spermatoza beyond the site of operation was discussed and the actual complementary method of contraception agreed on. It was emphasized that this must be used until two negative sperm counts had been received. Though these were initially requested at 12 and 16 weeks postoperatively the patient was told that complete azoospermia may take much longer to achieve. Time off from work in relation to the man's job was considered, and warning was given about the small incidence of infection and bleeding.

With this information the couple finally made their decision, and if they wished to proceed they and the doctor signed a consent form. They were told that "the absolute reliability of this method is unknown but it is the best we know." If there was any difficulty in making the decision discussion between the interviewing doctor and the surgeon took place in the clinic immediately, and subsequently with the general practitioner. In some cases the surgeon made the final decision after interviewing the couple himself. If there was a history of any genital abnormality or hernias the patient was examined by the surgeon during the first clinic visit.

Role of General Practitioner

Because of his knowledge of the whole family situation the general practitioner's agreement that vasectomy was desirable was regarded as essential before the operation was performed. Most patients were referred by their family doctor, usually at the patients' initial request. The general practitioner was also asked whether, so far as he knew, the couple were stable and happily married. On two occasions the general practitioner withheld his agreement. In two further instances the family doctor had a religious objection to sterilization, and he replaced the usual agreement form with a letter saying that there were no medical contraindications to the operation.

The Operation

The surgical team consisted of two general surgeons, three gynaecological surgeons, and one genitourinary surgeon. A theatre sister assisted and complete aseptic precautions were taken. Three operations were performed at each clinic session while other couples were being interviewed. Before the operation the surgeon considered fully the details on which the operation had initially been recommended at the time of interview.

Twenty-four hours before operation the patient shaved his scrotum. No preoperative medication was given. At operation the surgeon fixed the vas with the finger and thumb of one hand and local anaesthetic was injected into the skin and alongside the vas itself; 2 to 5 ml. of 1% lignocaine hydrochloride B.P. (without adrenaline) was used for the whole procedure. The skin was incised and the vas and its coverings were picked up with Poirer's forceps. A plane of cleavage was found immediately adjacent to the vas beneath the adherent vessels. Stripping the vas in this plane was bloodless and usually simple. Either one midline or two lateral incisions were made. The length of vas removed on each side was about 3-4 cm. (all were measured and recorded). The cut ends of the vasa were doubled back and ligated with catgut. In the first 100 patients the vasa were tied with thread. Haemostasis was achieved and two catgut stitches were placed in the skin wound. Dry gauze was placed over the incision and kept in place with stretch pants. Each operation lasted 15 to 20 minutes.

Care was taken that a conversation of interest to the patient was continued between him and the sister and the surgeon throughout the operation. The patient was warned that bruising might occur, that the effect of the local anaesthetic would wear off in about an hour, and that any subsequent pain could be controlled by aspirin and should diminish in intensity after 24 hours. He went home immediately after the operation, being asked to return in one week for postoperative follow-up.

Semen Analyses

Tests were originally asked for at 8, 10, and 12 weeks postoperatively, but, as one-third of the patients were still positive at 10 weeks, later semen analyses were requested at 12 and 16 weeks postoperatively. All slides were filed for reference. The operation was regarded as complete when two seminal analyses showed azoospermia at an interval of one month, and letters to this effect were sent to the patient and to his general practitioner.

Results

Interviews

Of the 390 discussions during the 20 months under review 330 were followed by operation, 26 men were awaiting operation, and 34 did not proceed to operation for the following reasons.

```
Advised to postpone decision as parents and children were very
    young (2 returned in 12 and 18 months for operation) ..      ..  13
Patients elected to postpone decision as method was too final (2
    returned in 6 and 7 months for operation)       ..      ..      7
Referred for tubal ligation      ..      ..      ..      ..      ..  6
Referred for hysterectomy      ..      ..      ..      ..      ..  1
General practitioner did not agree      ..      ..      ..      ..  2
Had vasectomy under National Health Service      ..      ..      ..  2
Emigrated      ..      ..      ..      ..      ..      ..      ..  1
Patient had a coronary thrombosis      ..      ..      ..      ..  1
Ex-prisoner moved away after release from prison      ..      ..  1
```

First 100 Interviews Preceding Operation

```
Age      ..      ..      ..  20-29      30-39      40-49      ≥50
    Husband      ..      ..      4      62      32      2
    Wife      ..      26      59      15      0
Years of marriage: 39 < 10 years; 55 10-19 years; 6 ` 20 years
Health ..      ..      ..  Well      Some Ill Health      Severe Illness
    Husband ..      ..      73      22      5
    Wife      ..      ..      71      19      10
Obstetric history: 57 normal; 26 some abnormality; 17 severe abnormality
Children per family: 43 had 1 or 2; 51 had 3 or 4; 6 had 5 to 9—total
    288 children
Pregnancies: 288 live births; 37 abortions; 1 termination
Unplanned pregnancies: 132 (40·5",.)
Patient's reasons for vasectomy:
```

```
Family large enough—cannot afford more or "cannot cope"
    with more      ..      ..      ..      ..      ..      ..      ..  56
Alternative methods unacceptable      ..      ..      ..      ..  53
Ill health of husband      ..      ..      ..      ..      ..      ..  4
Ill health of wife      ..      ..      ..      ..      ..      ..  36
Inherited defects of children      ..      ..      ..      ..      ..  3
Age ..      ..      ..      ..      ..      ..      ..      ..      ..  25
```

Three reasons were commonly given.

```
                              ┌ Sheath      ..      ..      ..      ..  91
                              │ Pill      ..      ..      ..      ..  54
                              │ Diaphragm      ..      ..      ..      ..  49
Previous contraceptives       │ Coitus interruptus      ..      ..  39
    used                      ┤ Pessaries          ⎫
                              │ Foam               ⎬      ..      ..  17
                              │ Rhythm method      ⎭
                              │ Intrauterine device      ..      ..  15
                              └ Complete abstinence      ..      ..  15
```

51 couples had tried three or more methods.

```
                          ┌ Offered but vasectomy preferred      ..  30
Female sterilization  ┤ Requested but refused (5 medically
                          │      contraindicated) ..      ..      ..  20
                          └ Patient had not requested      ..      ..  50
```

```
Coital frequency ┌ Twice or less per week      ..      ..      ..  45
                 └ Three times or more per week      ..      ..  55
```

Immediate Results of Operation

The patient returned after one week and asked about any pain or loss of time from work. Signs of infection and haematoma were noted.

Pain.—Most men did not find pain troublesome except when they had a large haematoma.

Time off Work.—330 patients: 80 were not recorded, though one had considerable time off as a result of infection, and 250 were recorded (no time off 168 or 1 day off 45 (85·2%); 2 days off 19; 3 days off 6; 7 days off 10; one operation performed in hospital, two on holiday; 28 days off 1 with a haematoma).

Infection.—There were no significant wound infections. Two haematomata became infected—one soon after operation, needing incision in hospital; one four weeks after operation which discharged spontaneously and healed completely. There were no persistent sinuses.

Haematomata.—At one week half the patients had no haematoma or bruising. Slight bruising or haematomata of 3 cm. diameter or less occurred in the remainder, except in 14 patients who had haematomata large enough to need further medical care. Two of these were admitted to hospital—one recorded above, and the other for observation. None were evacuated surgically. Some of these haematomata were thought to be infected and antibiotics were given outside the clinic, possibly unecessarily.

Hospital Admissions.—Five patients were admitted for elective operation: one combined with removal of an atrophic testicle, one because of associated bleeding disease, one because of extreme anxiety in the clinic, and two whose vasa were not palpable in the clinic. Three patients were admitted for postoperative complications; one for incision of an infected haematoma (see above), one for two days' observation of a large haematoma (see above), and one for a stitch in a bleeding scrotal incision.

Results of Semen Analysis

The term "completed" indicates two consecutive semen analyses showing azoospermia at one month's interval. Among the 330 patients under review analyses were not completed in 132, as insufficient time had elapsed since operation. Of the 198 in whom it could have been completed 172 had a complete operation and 26 did not.

Analysis of 172 Completed Operations.—Of 152 patients who sent in two specimens (both azoospermic) 24 completed 12 weeks, 102 18 weeks, 19 24 weeks, and 7 30 weeks postoperatively. The 26 patients who completed in 24 weeks or more delayed submitting specimens. Fourteen patients sent in one positive specimen (these patients completed between 18 and 32 weeks postoperatively). Four sent in two positive specimens (these patients completed between 21 and 28 weeks postoperatively). Two sent in five positive specimens (one patient completed 35 weeks and one 38 weeks postoperatively).

Analysis of the 26 Patients whose Operations were Not Completed.—Twenty defaulted in submitting specimens (12

71

submitted none). The other six patients submitted persistently positive specimens (three of these submitted such specimens up to 38 weeks postoperatively, then stopped. On recall to the clinic they reported that they were abstaining, and were recorded in the initial interview as having had poorly established sexual relationships before operation).

Yearly Follow-ups

The few patients who were interviewed a year after completion of the operation were satisfied and had no regrets. Semen analyses at this stage had all been negative. These follow-ups will be the subject of a further report.

Conclusion

The interest in male sterilization in the community is considerable, and the demand for the operation far outstrips the services available. Sterilization is a permanent, irreversible method of contraception, and the decision to use this method is based on consideration of factors affecting the whole family. Male and female sterilization are considered, but vasectomy is much preferred by most of the couples in this series because it is simple and the mother does not have to leave her family.

The operation can be carried out in the outpatient department under local anaesthesia with little or no time off work and a very low complication rate. Certain information and skills seem advisable before vasectomy is undertaken. The general practitioner is best able to assess family stability, the decision is taken only after consideration of other contraceptive methods, and surgical experience is needed even though the operation is a minor one.

The results reported above indicate that vasectomy is a simple, safe, aesthetic, efficient, and cheap method of achieving permanent family limitation.

We wish to thank the lay and nursing staff of the Family Planning Association who worked in the vasectomy clinic; to the pathologists and technicians who undertook the semen analyses; to the Board of Governors of the United Cardiff Hospitals for their permission to use the outpatient theatre and premises; and to the many people throughout Cardiff Royal Infirmary who co-operated so generously.

72

Vasectomy and Adverse Psychological Reactions

FREDERICK J. ZIEGLER, M.D.

SINCE the recent adverse publicity concerning ovulation suppressor contraception, there is reason to believe that there has been a major epidemic of unwanted pregnancies and, for many couples, an increase in requests for vasectomy as the most acceptable contraceptive option. A review of the evidence concerning possible psychological upset after vasectomy may therefore be timely. There have been several reports of psychiatric problems after and apparently related to vasectomy (1). Most questionnaire surveys made of couples after vasectomy report almost complete satisfaction with the procedure as a contraceptive method (2). In a follow-up study of some patients who had help in arranging their vasectomy from the Association for Voluntary Sterilization, it was concluded that "these men and their friends and their relatives hold stereotyped attitudes equating vasectomy with being castrated and made inferior, and that the good results indicate adequate coping with the psychological factors by a large majority of the respondents" (3). A prospective noncontrolled study by questionnaire and psychological testing (the Minnesota Multiphasic Personality Inventory) of 35 men again indicated stated satisfaction with the procedure on the questionnaire but showed psychological test evidence of emotional upset 1 to 1½ years postoperatively (4). Fifteen of these subjects showed negative changes, but two showed evidence of improvement. The men who showed the adverse changes tended to have shown preoperative test evidence of hypochondriasis or concerns about their masculinity. In the study just mentioned earlier (3), it was concluded that "the strongest contraindication for a vasectomy is disagreement with one's wife over its advisability."

In another longitudinal prospective study, 37 men and their wives were seen for psychiatric interviews and psychological testing before vasectomy and were followed-up periodically with repeat testing, interviewing, and questionnaires over a 4-year period. They

73

were compared with 22 couples who elected ovulation-suppressor contraception and were similarly studied over the same period of time (5). After 2 years the men who had obtained vasectomy and their wives were somewhat more psychologically upset than the control couples and somewhat less happy with their marriages. Some compensatory stereotyped and exaggerated masculine behavior was found in many of these men even after 4 years, suggesting that vasectomy is reacted to by most subjects and their wives as if the operation had "demasculinizing potential." At the end of 4 years, however, there was no more evidence of psychologic upset or marital problems in the vasectomy group than in the control group, lending support to the conclusion of the study cited above (3) that the psychological problems associated with vasectomy are such that most men can cope with them adequately after a time. It seemed very likely that the intensive interviewing of both vasectomy and ovulation-suppressor couples was relatively effective in aborting or defusing the possible psychological complications of vasectomy. When vasectomy was elected in part because of the frigidity of the wife or premature ejaculation of the husband, such problems did not tend to improve (6), so vasectomy does not seem indicated for specific sexual problems.

It would appear then that psychological problems can occur in men after vasectomy and in their wives, that such reactions are seldom but occasionally of an extensive degree, that such upset is not ordinarily attributed to the vasectomy by the man or his wife and satisfaction with vasectomy is generally reported, and that psychologic upset associated with vasectomy apparently can usually be aborted by psychiatric interviewing and presumably by discussions with an informed counselor. The fact that vasovasostomy (reversal of vasectomy) can now be performed successfully by at least several urologists in a very high percentage (perhaps over 90%) of men is useful information to patients and prospective patients for minimizing the psychological impact of the procedure. With appropriate counseling vasectomy may at this time be an attractive (relative to the other currently available options) contraceptive method for families who have the desired number of children, in which husband and wife are both agreed on the procedure, and in which the husband is not unusually hypochondriacal or concerned about his masculinity.

References

1. JOHNSON MD: Social and psychological effects of vasectomy. *Amer J Psychiat* 121:482-486, 1964

2. LANDIS JT, POFFENBERGER T: The marital and sexual adjustment of 330 couples who chose vasectomy as a form of birth control. *J Marriage Family* 27:57-58, 1965
3. FERBER S, TIETZE C, LEWIT S: Men with vasectomies: a study of medical, sexual, and psychosocial changes. *Psychosom Med* 29:354-366, 1967
4. RODGERS DA, ZIEGLER FJ, ALTROOCHI J, et al: A longitudinal study of the psycho-social effects of vasectomy. *J Marriage Family* 27:59-64, 1965
5. ZIEGLER FJ, RODGERS DA, PRENTISS RJ: Psychosocial response to vasectomy. *Arch Gen Psychiat (Chicago)* 21:46-54, 1969
6. RODGERS DA, ZIEGLER FJ: Changes in sexual behavior consequent to use of noncoital procedures of contraception. *Psychosom Med* 30:495-505, 1968

75

Is Sterilization the Answer?

Moni Nag

The lamentable lack of knowledge about the consequence of sterilization perhaps accounts for the strong opposition to it by the Cornell students and faculty when they were polled recently on various methods of birth control ("Population control, sterilization, and ignorance," 23 Jan., p. 337). Fifty-two percent of males and sixty-one percent of females said they would *never* undergo sterilization, even after having had the desired number of children. About one-half favored the oral contraceptives over all other available means. Even a large proportion of biology students confessed ignorance or doubt about the well-established fact that vasectomy does not abolish the ability to ejaculate. In India about 5 million vasectomy operations have been performed since 1956 and complaints about any adverse effect of the operation on the sexual function of the sterilized men have been almost absent.

The results obtained at Cornell certainly emphasize the need for very comprehensive sex education including physiology of reproduction and methods of birth control. The valiant efforts of SIECUS (Sex Information and Educational Council of the U.S.) to introduce sex education in the schools have recently been opposed by a few conservative groups such as the John Birch Society. It needs the active support of scientists and other open-minded persons so that everybody can acquire adequate knowledge of sex and its related aspects in life. Only then can we expect adults to make a more intelligent choice of the method of family planning or limitation. If this is true for a highly literate society as in the United States, it is much more true for other societies with lower literacy levels.

Psychological Aspects of Vasectomy

HELEN WOLFERS, B.SC.

Introduction

The demand for contraceptive sterilization of men is rising
steeply in both the U.S and the U.K., and the increased concern over side effects of contraceptive pills will further accel-
erate this demand. As a surgical procedure this operation has
proved safe and reliable over a period approaching 70 years.
It has, however, been established that, whereas 2% of normal
men have circulating antibodies against their own sperm, they
are present in 30% of vasectomized men (Rumke and
Hellinga, 1959; Phadke and Padukone, 1964). While at
present this appears to be of academic interest only, the possibility of autoimmune conditions developing as a remote
sequel to vasectomy cannot be entirely dismissed. One report
has appeared (Roberts, 1968) recording a few cases which
might be of this nature.

As a contraceptive measure the irreversibility of the operation is its most serious defect. Some encouraging success,
however, has been reported by various doctors in reversing
the operation surgically (Dorsey, 1957; Roland, 1961). But
even successful restoration of patency does not guarantee
restoration of fecundity, for most men with anti-sperm
antibodies are rendered sterile by this factor, and many of

77

the possible psychological problems at present associated with vasectomy may well be due to its present practical irreversibility.

Psychological Implications of Vasectomy

Quite apart from the conscious regrets which unforeseen circumstances may cause the individual who can no longer father children, the concept of permanent sterility itself has in all probability profound emotional significance for the male in a patriarchal society. Morris (1967) built up a convincing theory concerning the adaptation of man's behavioural patterns to serve his unique paternal role in the animal kingdom. Irrational and unconsciously motivated behaviour primarily patterned to protect the young he begets persists redundantly in modern man. The removal of his ability to produce the young (or impregnate the mate) he still unconsciously acts to protect must inevitably affect all men on some level, no matter how deeply unconscious.

Erikson (1954) and Johnson (1964a) detailed case studies of vasectomized men encountered in their psychiatric practices. The finding of six such men in Erikson's own analytic practice suggests a far higher proportion of vasectomized men to be found in psychiatric clinics than in the population at large. Nevertheless, this high incidence is not necessarily evidence of any causal connexion between vasectomy and psychiatric illness. The only controlled experiment involving preoperative and postoperative psychological testing has produced tentative findings which do indeed indicate that submission to vasectomy may itself be indicative of personality disorder and, in turn, also lead to increased psychological disturbance (Rogers, Ziegler, Altrocchi, and Levy, 1965). In the past, however, psychological studies of the effects of vasectomy have necessarily had to deal with highly self-selected samples. So long as vasectomy remained an obscure contraceptive practice, men with specialized requirements, either psychological or physical, would be expected to be disproportionately represented among those who actively sought out or were invited to submit to this procedure.

The studies so far reported on this subject, with the exception of the study by Rogers et al. (1965), have been of two types.

(1) Questionnaire surveys (Garrison and Gamble, 1950; Dandekar, 1963; Landis and Poffenberger, 1965; Ferber, Tietze, and Lewit, 1967; Simon Population Trust, 1969), which ask men themselves to evaluate their sex lives and marital and other personal relations before and after the operation, invariably indicate that the vast majority would choose to have the operation again if the circumstances arose

(or would recommend it to others or have no regrets at having had it). A very small proportion ranging from 1 to 3% have suffered some deterioration in their sexual lives, and, also invariably, the percentage who would have the operation again exceeds the percentage who have not suffered sexual damage from it, leaving a small proportion of men who claim that they would have the operation again despite sexual deterioration. It is interesting that most authors have failed to mention this persistent paradox. This raises the suspicion of unconscious motivation on their part to demonstrate the benefits of vasectomy and overlook its problems (Johnson, 1964b).

(2) Case histories of psychiatric patients who have had vasectomies. Those psychiatrists who have written on the subject have been unanimous in condemning vasectomy as a psychologically dangerous procedure.

Rosen (1954) stated bluntly that sterilizing operations "are *never* performed merely as contraceptive measures." Erikson (1954) stated that vasectomy, though often requested as a contraceptive measure, seldom is. It is rather a means for emotionally sick women to castrate their husbands, an act of masochism, or an unconscious abortion. He quotes colloquialisms, such as the "spayed bitch" and the "dumb ox" compared with the "spirited stallion" and the "virile man," as evidence for universal unconscious attitudes of human beings to fertility. A capon or steer is only meat, but a rooster and bull are living creatures. Erikson's point is a fallacious one, however. He argues that the preservation of gender is a biological necessity and any wilful destruction thereof inevitably leads to a lowering of self-esteem. But there is neither loss of virility nor of gender involved in vasectomy; Erikson is confusing vasectomy with castration, equating sterility with the loss of gender, and confounding infertility with impotence in animals. His oversight is in itself of special significance, as one may readily accept that if so highly educated a man, a doctor and psychiatrist himself, can unconsciously omit so fundamental a distinction of which he is undoubtedly consciously aware, the two procedures, though consciously distinct, or even when made so by education, will nevertheless always remain unconsciously equivalent to some extent for most of mankind.

Unreal as Erikson's argument is, in fact, the unconscious equating of vasectomy with castration may nevertheless be an unavoidable reality. Evidence of this has been demonstrated by Ziegler, Rogers, and Kriegsman (1965). Using projective tests they found that the vasectomized man is seen as emasculated. Behaviour too was affected after vasectomy in that activities associated with sex roles, such as child-rearing and household chores, assume new dimensions in family relations. They found adverse changes in marital relations, as the operation appeared to give rise to scrutiny of the man by himself and by others for evidence of unmasculine behaviour. Perhaps because of oedipal anxieties and unconscious fears of genital mutilation vasectomy seems to threaten men's sense of masculinity.

Johnson (1964a), again from observation of psychiatric patients who had previously had vasectomies for contraceptive purposes, concluded that "the operation was not as innocuous as commonly believed" and that failure to limit family size by the conventional methods could of itself reflect other unnoticed problems in the marriage, which then became centred on the operation. But these reports, like those of Erikson, are based on observations of psychologically disturbed people only.

Hostility

Antagonism Among Researchers

Vasectomy is a highly emotional issue to several groups in the community with (real or imaginary) conflicting interests. On the one hand, one can appreciate the zeal it has aroused in family planning circles as a safe, simple, and reliable form of permanent contraception. On the other hand, it involves issues of the most fundamental nature to psychoanalysis. And still again, it is the first attempt to engage the male in biological (as opposed to physical) forms of contraception which may involve pain and risk.

The polarization of this research into camps of those in favour and those against is therefore not surprising. It has led to animated criticisms of one by the other. O'Connor (1950), attacking the survey method, wrote: "Psychic and emotional effects of vasectomy are much greater and more deeply rooted than an analysis of such factors as the 'effect on libido,' 'postorgasmal symptoms' and 'frequency of intercourse' would indicate." He continued that making a man "safe sexually" (a revealingly aggressive equivalent for infertile) has often resulted in marital infidelity, domestic discord, separation, and divorce. This increase in marital infidelity has not been found in survey-type studies, despite frequent attention to it, and it is a pity that O'Connor has not published his figures on this question and divorce rates from his records.

Bass and Laidlaw, respectively president and vice-president of the Human Betterment Association for Voluntary Sterilization, "refuted" such criticisms of vasectomy on the grounds that the "birthquake" is the greatest problem facing the world today and that dwelling on the reports of possible psychological ill effects of so valuable a contraceptive procedure is not justifiable in the face of such an enormous human calamity (Laidlaw and Bass, 1964). Such arguments, however, are not valid (even if acceptable on ethical grounds), because a contraceptive method with harmful side effects released on large sections of a population will ultimately do more to retard than advance the cause of family planning.

80

Aggressive Use of Vasectomy

The antagonism met with in this field has extended recently beyond the range of research workers, doctors, and psychiatrists to a battle between the sexes. Quite apart from the aggressive use of vasectomy by husband against wife, or wife against husband (see Erikson, 1954; Johnson, 1964a; Ziegler et al., 1965; and this study), the lay press and the public in general have of late taken to discussing the issue of whose responsibility contraception is or ought to be. The recently published Family Planning Association poster in Britain depicting a pregnant man over a caption which reads "Would you be more careful if it was you that got pregnant?" illustrates this point.

Johnson (1964a) stated that a "still unexplored area [of vasectomy] concerns the stress that may be involved in . . . the performance of a surgical procedure on one person (husband) for the benefit of another (wife)." In the male mind (and, for all we know, in the female mind too) an unwanted pregnancy is still the woman's misfortune alone, and a great deal of unconscious resistance to the concept of male sterilization can be expected from this source.

Johnson further commented "that a major problem with vasectomy is the ease with which it can be . . . used to treat the *wrong* member of the family. Among our cases the overworked, overfertile housewife seems to be a more suitable candidate for sterilization than does her husband." The aggressive nature of such reports gives cause for concern that the intricate involvement of infantile psychological phenomena may be a complicating issue, not only for the subject but also for the student of vasectomy.

Ziegler et al. (1965) reported that some husbands in their study appeared to treat the vasectomy as a highly valued pawn in a sub rosa bargaining procedure, so that they reacted postoperatively as though they had made a great sacrifice for the marriage and no longer needed to be so considerate of their wives.

Present Investigation

We recently concluded a study in Swindon (Wilts.) in which 95 men who had undergone contraceptive vasectomy operations at the Simon Trust Clinic were sent questionnaires. No questions relating to sexual or marital adjustment were asked, but patients who believed that they had encountered such problems as a result of the operation were asked to request an appointment with a visiting psychologist.

Eighty-two men returned their forms, and of these seven requested appointments. Three others were also contacted to investigate comments made in answer to the question "Have you had any ill effects arising out of the operation?" In these cases the comments indicated psychological impairment. Thus

81

when offered the opportunity of personal interview with a professional 10 (12%) out of 82 signalled some psychological problem arising from the operation, compared with previous findings of 1-3%, in pure questionnaire surveys.

Of the seven couples who sought interviews only three were unaware of any physical or psychological problem in their sexual lives before the operation. No causal connexion between their vasectomies and the ensuing sexual problem is provable in the absence of prolonged psychoanalytic investigation (and even this would not be conclusive). The implication from the coincidence in time is that the operation did give rise to (or at least trigger) the ensuing disability, and, in the absence of evidence to the contrary, this must be accepted. All three couples suffered serious physical sexual deterioration involving complete impotence, vaginismus, and persistent premature ejaculation.

Three of the remaining four cases had pre-existing sexual problems: premature ejaculation, declining potency, or frigidity (in the wife). In none of these cases was the vasectomy at all successful in alleviating the sexual disability. In fact, two of these three couples believed that their symptoms had been made worse. The remaining patient, now suffering from depression and fear of impotence, had a long history of neurotic instability. Three other respondents indicated that they had suffered sexually or psychologically since the time of the operation, but they did not request appointments. In answer to the question "Have you had any ill effects arising out of the operation?" their replies suggested relative impotence, depression, and an episode of impotence after the operation.

Comparison of the demographic and social variables for the subgroup with psychological or sexual problems with those of the sample in general showed no significant differences. Of the seven couples who requested special interviews, however, five had histories of marital, sexual, or psychological instability. Without preoperative investigations and depth interviewing of the sample as a whole, no comparisons of these characteristics between this subsample and the larger group are possible, but the proportion is very high (70%), and it is reasonable to assume that histories of pre-existing marital, sexual, or psychological instability should be taken as a contraindication to vasectomy. In four of these five cases with pre-existing instability it appears unlikely that the operation has been responsible for anything more than the acceleration of a pre-existing process.

Similarly, Ferber et al. (1967) found that the three (out of 73) men who stated that they were less satisfied with their sexual lives after the operation each had a pre-existing potency problem which was aggravated after the operation. Probably had these men not undergone vasectomy some other life event would have served the purpose equally well.

It appears that the fear of impregnating the wife with an unwanted baby may have been serving a defensive purpose in

82

some of these cases by explaining the sexual problem for the couple. Removal of this fear would then be expected to result, as it did, in an aggravation of the problem, which obviously was not due to fear of pregnancy. Nevertheless, this is not evidence (and there is as yet no evidence to hand) that in cases in which the fear of pregnancy is the real underlying cause of sexual malfunctioning vasectomy is not an effective remedy. It is a defect of this study, as of all previous studies with the exception of that of Rogers *et al.* (1965), that the possibility of demonstrating salutary effects on pre-existing sexual problems has been excluded in the study design.

The three couples who claimed to have no pre-existing sexual problem are of paramount importance in this study, as here we have most reason to suspect that the vasectomy has been instrumental in initiating the sexual and psychological damage. The depth interviews revealed possible psychoanalytic explanations of the bad outcomes for two of the men.

One patient exhibited an unconscious hostility towards his wife which seems to have existed since the beginning of the marriage. He resented her lack of time and concern for their three children. Their sexual life was described by both as very good before the operation. Possibly the resulting impotence was an unconscious punishment of the wife by the husband which effectively said "if no more children, then no more pleasure." The operation had been undergone on their doctor's advice for the wife's sake, as further pregnancies or a female sterilization would have been detrimental to her health. Johnson's point that the psychological effects of an operation performed on one person for the benefit of another are as yet an unexplored phenomenon appears relevant to this case.

Another couple had both been married before. The wife was extremely unhappy with her first husband and had ascribed her frigidity to her dislike of him. Sexually the second marriage had been extremely successful until the operation, which was followed by vaginismus in the wife. We are led to suspect that she had failed to mature sexually, probably owing to faulty psychosexual development in the formative years of early childhood, which had resulted in deep-rooted feelings of guilt over sexual enjoyment. With the removal of the "bad man" by divorce, followed by the removal of the "justification" of procreation for sexual intercourse by vasectomy, vaginismus became the only line of defence left to her.

In the remaining case (premature ejaculation) no explanation for the outcome can be offered from the information available. The possibility of this being a physical rather than a psychological outcome cannot be discounted.

Paradoxical Answers

As in all other survey studies of vasectomy, it was found in this investigation that most of the men (or couples) who

83

believe themselves to have suffered sexually and psychologically from the operation nevertheless do not regret having had the operation. In view of the fact that there is a variety of other safe and reliable methods of contraception available to them, entailing less serious side effects in their particular circumstances, these statements appear paradoxical and require clarification. Ziegler et al. (1965) offered an explanation in terms of dissonance reduction; the individual having taken an irrevocable step has a need to convince himself that what he has done was in his best interest. This argument may also throw some light on the widespread readiness of vasectomized men to recommend the operation to others. The Simon Population Trust (1969), for example, found that 99% of men would recommend the operation, despite the fact that 5% reported a deterioration in the "harmony of marriage." Since we look for confirmation of reality in the opinions of others, the need to convince ourselves is served also by convincing others. Furthermore, there is a sense of comfort in numbers, and there may well be a need for vasectomized men in Western countries, where the operation is still relatively rare, to proselytize.

Apart from dissonance reduction, overcompensation is also involved in this reaction. This phenomenon is discussed by Ferber et al. (1967) (though not in relation to the paradoxical findings of their survey). Accepting that vasectomy must invariably lead to some lowering of self-esteem (see above), all men who have experienced it will require to adjust to a changed self-image in order to cope successfully with its psychological effects. To do this they appear to use a sense of increased mastery over their own destinies and of relief at having no further decision to make. It is this process of overcompensation which leads to exaggerated reports of satisfaction with the operation from most couples, and it is even more vital to men who have suffered sexual impairment from vasectomy than to those who have not.

Conclusion

The collection of data by questionnaire surveys is too simple a procedure to assess reliably the psychosocial and sexual effects of contraceptive vasectomy. Motivated by the possibility of receiving help with their problems a much higher proportion of respondents stated that sexual inadequacies had led them to seek the operation and had (in their own opinions) resulted from it than has hitherto been found by traditional survey methods. The findings of this study indicate that some screening of applicants for contraceptive vasectomy is required, and it is tentatively suggested that men with marital, psychological, or sexual problems should be dissuaded from this form of contraception.

Further study is required, however, to determine whether the operation is successful in curing some types of psycho-

84

sexual disorders, as any possible cures which may have followed contraceptive vasectomy have epistemologically been excluded in all studies (with one exception) so far.

I am indebted to Mr. Munro, of the Simon Trust Clinic in Swindon, whose co-operation made this study possible; to Mrs. Paine, his secretary, for her help in the organization of it; and to the Ministry of Overseas Development for financing the research.

REFERENCES

Dandekar, K. (1963). *Artha Vijnana*, **5**, 212.

Dorsey, J. W. (1957). *Journal of the International College of Surgeons*, **27**, 453.

Erikson, M. H. (1954). In *Therapeutic Abortion*, ed. H. Rosen, p. 57. New York, Julian Press.

Ferber, A. S., Tietze, C., and Lewit, S. (1967). *Psychosomatic Medicine*, **29**, 354.

Garrison, P. L., and Gamble, C. J. (1950). *Journal of the American Medical Association*, **144**, 293.

Johnson, M. H. (1964a). *American Journal of Psychiatry*, **121**, 482.

Johnson, M. H. (1964b). *Issues in Current Medical Practice*, **1**, No. 10.

Laidlaw, R. W., and Bass, M. S. (1964). *American Journal of Psychiatry*, **120**, 1176.

Landis, J. T., and Poffenberger, T. (1965). *Journal of Marriage and the Family*, **27**, 57.

Morris, D. (1967). *The Naked Ape*. London, Cape.

O'Connor, V. J. (1950). *Journal of the American Medical Association*, **144**, 1502.

Phadke, A. M., and Padukone, K. (1964). *Journal of Reproduction and Fertility*, **7**, 163.

Roberts, H. J. (1968). *Journal of the American Geriatrics Society*, **16**, 267.

Rogers, D. A., Ziegler, F. J., Altrocchi, J., and Levy, N. (1965). *Journal of Marriage and the Family*, **27**, 59.

Roland, S. I. (1961). *Fertility and Sterility*, **12**, 191.

Rosen, H. (editor) (1954). *Therapeutic Abortion*, p. 33. New York, Julian Press.

Rumke, P., and Hellinga, G. (1959). *American Journal of Clinical Pathology*, **32**, 357.

Simon Population Trust (1969). *Vasectomy: Follow-up of a Thousand Cases*. Cambridge, Simon Population Trust.

Ziegler, F. J., Rogers, D. A., and Kriegsman, S. A. (1965). Effect of vasectomy on psychological functioning. Paper presented at the annual meeting (May) of the American Psychosomatic Society, Philadelphia, U.S.A.

85

Voluntary Sterilisation in the Male

D. Urquhart-Hay FRCS FRACS

INTRODUCTION

In spite of considerable discussion of this problem over the last few years, there is still much confusion amongst the medical profession as to whether male sterilisation for reasons of contraceptive convenience is lawful or not. Many still believe that it is illegal to sterilise a male for reasons other than to protect his physical or mental health. A few believe that it is lawful. The majority are not certain and while prepared to accept it as an ethical procedure, prefer to occupy themselves in less controversial areas. In fact, although prior to 1960 the Medical Defence Society discouraged the procedure, it has never ever been illegal, and since that date there has been a considerable change in legal thinking to the point that now it is generally accepted the operation is lawful provided the full and valid consent of the person is obtained.

There can be little doubt that vasectomy is the most effective method of contraception that we have. It is a minor procedure, permanent, and effective. It has no effect on potency or libido, and is free from psychological sequelae. Compare this with the major procedure of tubal ligation in the female with a possible morbidity rate and failure rate as high as four percent. The "pill" even if taken regularly, is not without its problems. The number of cases of depression, nausea, weight gain, irritability, loss of libido, etc., are well known, and its long term effects are not yet fully appreciated. Intra-uterine devices have a high extrusion rate, and are also responsible for bleeding, discomfort, occasional infection, and even ectopic pregnancies. Those who are prepared to accept the inconvenience and aesthetic deficiencies of the cervical cap, douching, and condoms, must be prepared to accept an even higher failure rate. I think most people would accept that at the present state of our knowledge, vasectomy is the most simple, direct and effective method of contraception available. Why then, does this confusion exist as to whether the operation is lawful or not?

HISTORICAL ASPECTS

It all goes back to the thirteenth century when any person who injured or maimed a man could be charged with the indictable trespass of maim or mayhem. Maim at that time was defined as an injury which resulted in a man being rendered less able to defend himself; the reason for this trespass was to discourage wastage of manpower and thus enable the king to maintain a standing army. Consent was no defence. Castration would constitute a maim. This common law has stuck with us over the centuries, and up until 1960 it was still believed by lawyers that to sterilise a male would lead to the surgeon exposing himself to legal proceedings. In fact in 1949 three medical defence organisations in England sought the opinion of legal counsel upon whether sterilisation of a male or female was legal and if so, in what circumstances. Counsel gave an opinion that sterilisation on eugenic grounds was illegal, unless there were valid therapeutic reasons. This seemed to establish the illegality of sterilisation. However, in 1960 further opinion was sought. A contrary view was now expressed and published in the Annual Report of the Medical Defence Union, 1961, namely: "Sterilisation is not unlawful whether it is performed on therapeutic or eugenic grounds or for other reasons, provided there is full and valid consent to do the operation by the patient concerned".

In 1965 an organisation called the Simon Population Trust was established in England to promote voluntary sterilisation for family welfare, and largely through their influence and the work of Blacker and Jackson (1966) much attention has been focused on this problem. Their enquiries led them to conclude that voluntary sterilisation carried out in good faith for adequate reasons and with the written consent of both spouses was not illegal.

In 1966 Addison, secretary of the Medical Defence Union, reaffirmed the opinion expressed by counsel in 1961, but reminded the profession that this opinion was not based on any stable judicial authority as it had never been tested in the courts, but he pointed out that "members of the union may rest assured that if, as the result of the performance of an operation for primary sterilisation, they find themselves in any sort of medico-legal difficulty, they can count on the full support of the union ".

Thus, with the assurance of a leading legal counsel that the operation was lawful, the establishment of an influential society to promote the operation, and the assurance of the Medical Defence Society that they would lend their full support in protecting any surgeon who found himself the subject of a prosecution, the operation of vasectomy became not only lawful but respectable.

SURGICAL TECHNIQUE

The operation itself is a minor one, and to the urologist who has been used to the technique of tying the vasa during the operation of prostatectomy, it will present few problems. It is preferable to do these cases under general anaesthesia in hospital on a day-stay basis. I am against the practice of operating under local anaesthesia in the consulting room; bleeding is occasionally a problem, and in those cases where the vas slips back into the wound and re-exploration is necessary, local anaesthesia can be an embarrassment. The operation is done through two small incisions in the upper scrotum, the vas is exteriorised and a one-inch segment excised and the residual ends of the vas ligated with plain catgut. Hanley (1968) has recently drawn attention to the rare occurrence of regeneration of the vas and has suggested a modification of the technique to prevent this. The patient generally rests at home on the following day and is fit to resume full duties on the third day.

It is important to explain to both husband and wife that the male is not sterile for about two to three months after the operation, and that during this time they must continue to use their usual contraceptive technique. This delay is due to the time taken to deplete the store of sperms contained in the seminal vesicles, and it is related to the frequency of coitus, the more frequently intercourse takes place the quicker the sperm depletion. It is my practice to collect a specimen of semen (by condom or masturbation) at two to three months following operation, and not until there is a total absence of sperms in the semen pronounce the person sterile. In spite of the fact that fertility is unlikely with a sperm count under twenty millions per cubic millimetre, one sperm, theoretically, can fertilise an ovum, and although one may have to wait an extra three or four weeks to achieve azoospermia, the knowledge is reassuring to the surgeon and couple alike. Provided contraceptive precautions are taken during this period, coitus can be resumed as soon after the operation as the patient prefers. A few complain of discomfort in the incision

88

on ejaculation, but this is unusual. Many patients are puzzled as to what happens to the sperms following this operation, and ask whether their testicles will swell or not. One can reassure them that although sperm production continues unabated, they are phagocytosed in the epididymes and no tension pains occur. Indeed the effect of this operation on the testis is negligible, and there is no loss of weight or alteration in testicular histology.

SUITABILITY OF CASES

The usual person referred for vasectomy is a married male in his thirties or forties, with two to three children, whose wife has found the "pill" unsuitable for various reasons—weight gain, irritability, or loss of libido. Other methods of contraception are usually unacceptable. The couple are usually adamant that they have enough children, and that further children would be disastrous for socio-economic reasons. They have usually discussed the problem fully between themselves and with their practitioner. Frequently the wives are anxious that it may alter their husband's sexual potency, and upset him psychologically—reassurance readily allays such fears. It is important to interview both husband and wife together, so that one can assess the couple and see that they fully understand the nature of their request. One should point out that although the operation is permanent, a re-anastomosis can always be attempted with a success rate of about 50 percent. It is essential to emphasise that it takes two to three months before the male is rendered sterile. I have both husband and wife sign a statement which I witness, confirming that they fully understand the nature and effect of the operation, and that they give me their consent to have it carried out on the husband. Consent on the part of the patient is a necessary legal safeguard in any operation to protect the surgeon; the wife's signature in this case is to protect the husband from a divorce suit on the grounds of constructive desertion. The view has also been expressed (although the issue has never been tested in the courts) that both the husband and wife might have a right of action in damages against the surgeon who sterilised one spouse either without the consent of, or in the face of a positive prohibition, by the other. In a divorce case arising out of a vasectomy *Bravery v Bravery* (1954) the Court of Appeal said: "We find it difficult to believe that any surgeon, a member of an honourable profession, would perform an operation of this kind on a young man unless he was first satisfied that the wife consented ".

It is my practice then, to carry out a vasectomy for any couple, who for socio-economic reasons wish to limit their family, or who for reasons of contraceptive convenience wish to have it done. They must be a stable and happily married couple, generally with a family, who are prepared to discuss their problem fully with me and give me their written permission to operate and assurance that they understand the nature of their request.

I would not limit the operation to married males, but I would be very cautious in operating on single males unless the reasons were ethically acceptable. One must probe carefully for a history of neurosis or psychosis, as subsequent ailments may easily be attributed to the vasectomy itself. Although the operation is lawful, one must be careful not to bring discredit to the profession by operating in a case in which the ethics of so doing are questionable, and likely to be judged as unacceptable by contemporary moral standards. If there is any doubt as to the suitability or otherwise of the case, a second medical opinion should always be sought.

DISCUSSION

But in spite of assurances that vasectomy is not unlawful, many surgeons still find the situation uncomfortable. They have no objections to the procedure on ethical grounds, but are frightened by the law. It comforts them little that the defence societies will come to their aid in the unlikely event of their being prosecuted, and they would sooner occupy themselves with less controversial operations. Because of this, an editorial in the *British Medical Journal* (1968) recently suggested that the matter should be settled either by having a test case in the courts, or else changing the law. Reaction to this suggestion was considerable. To provide a test case for the courts would be difficult, and in spite of the fact that Mr James Stirling QC, the barrister who in 1961 pronounced that male sterilisation is lawful, has since been elevated to the bench, a jury might come to the wrong decision. Even if the right decision were made, it might be too rigid and freeze the legal situation, as did the *Bourne* case in abortion law reform. Antagonists of this editorial view also point out that since the operation was declared lawful in 1961 there have been many thousands of vasectomies carried out in England, and no case has ever been challenged or prosecuted by the courts.

The suggestion that legislation be enacted by Parliament has also been sharply criticised. The Abortion Act does not inspire confidence in the ability of Parliament to grapple with medical subjects, and anyway most authorities regard the procedure as lawful already without recourse to legislation.

The benefits of male sterilisation have been recognised by many countries. The American Association for Voluntary Sterilisation Incorporated, with similar safeguards as the Simon Population Trust, accounts for one hundred thousand sterilisations per year. A similar organisation in Canada, the Parents' Information Bureau, has been established, and again promotes vasectomies for medico-social reasons. In India with a rocketing population, of approximately twelve million per year, a target of two million vasectomies per year has been set. Similar sterilisation policies are being developed in other Asian countries, namely, Pakistan, Korea, Taiwan, and even mainland China.

In New Zealand there seems little doubt that the public are now and possibly have always been happy to accept this sterilising procedure on the male. After all, a sensible, mature man can appreciate the significance and consequences of permanent sterilisation as well as his medical adviser. As Haynes (1967) pointed out, it is "nauseatingly hypocritical to find legal and moral objections to vasectomy in the so-called advanced countries, but to extol its use in under-developed areas".

The doctor's reluctance to recommend and perform this operation has been based on his ignorance and fear of the law. There is little doubt that provided the safeguards recommended by the Medical Defence Society are adhered to, the procedure of male sterilisation for reasons of contraceptive convenience is lawful.

REFERENCES

Addison, P. H. (1966). Sterilisation and the law. Br. med. J., 1, 1597.

Blacker, C. P. and Jackson, L. N. (1966). Voluntary sterilisation for family welfare. Lancet 1, 971-974.

Bravery v Bravery (1954). 1, W.L.R., 1167.

Editorial (1968). Voluntary sterilisation in the male. Br. med. J., 2, 508.

Haynes, W. S. (1967). Vasectomy. Med. J. Aust., 1, 1045-1048.

Hanley, H. G. (1968). Vasectomy for voluntary male sterilisation. Lancet 2, 207-209.

Medico-legal Implications of Vasectomy

By I. F. POTTS, M.S., F.R.C.S., F.R.A.C.S.

As there has never been a test case in Australia, legal opinions regarding vasectomy are speculative and qualified. A surgeon who undertakes vasectomy may have charges brought against him as a criminal action for alleged illegal operation or criminal assault or as a civil action on charges of assault or negligence. The consensus of opinion is that neither criminal nor civil action would succeed against the attending surgeon as long as certain agreed forms of consent had been obtained and the surgeon acted in a professional manner.

It is most strongly recommended that any surgeon who intends to carry out vasectomy should take great care to attend to the following points in all cases. Signed consent forms should be obtained from both the husband and the wife, who should be interviewed together. The operation and the effects of the operation should be explained in detail and notes to this effect should be entered on the case records which should include the accurate notation of all interviews. Excised specimens of each vas deferens should be sent for pathological examination to confirm that the vas has in fact been removed from each side. The surgeon should have a second medical opinion in confirmation of the propriety of the operation. It should be emphasised to the patient and his wife that the state of sterility awaits the result of serial semen analyses of which at least two should show azoospermia. If there is doubt about the maturity, mentality or psychological stability of the patient, then the surgeon should refuse to undertake the operation of vasectomy.

VASECTOMY FOR VOLUNTARY MALE
STERILISATION

Philip M. Alderman

Mr. Hanley's article (July 27, p. 207) effectively points out the risks of vasectomy, as well as its advantages. He rightly emphasises that there is a failure and morbidity rate, which has likewise been my own experience in just over 2000 cases in the past six years. However, Mr. Hanley does not mention what these rates have been in his own experience, or what might be acceptable. Without this information it would be difficult to assess one's own results. It would be useful to know, for example, the total number of vasectomies performed, the number of failures involved, and the number and types of complications. For those contemplating or performing vasectomies I report here my own experience.

Up to Aug. 3, 1968, I had performed 1923 vasectomies, of which 19 were failures—a failure-rate of 0·98%. If one subtracts 6 failures, resulting from an experimental series of 10 patients in the group on whom only vas ligation was performed, the failure rate drops to 0·68%. Only 2 cases came to my attention in which a haematoma was a postoperative complication, and there were 3 scrotal abscesses. All operations were performed under local anaesthesia in my office, suggesting that there may be no advantage in putting patients to the trouble and expense of a general anaesthetic in order to lessen the risk of such complications.

In view of the foregoing, and contrary to Mr. Hanley's caveats, it may be of interest that I make no effort to overlap the severed vas ends, to fold the ends back, or to separate them in different tissue planes. The procedure is simple and safe enough for any competent general practitioner to perform in his office, and consists merely of removing about 1·5 cm. of vas between two clamps and carefully tying off the ends with chromic suture. That simple division alone, even without ligature, can produce sterility is well illustrated by the 5 cases of sterility mentioned by Mr. Hanley following accidental surgical injury. Careful ligation of the vas ends, however, is recommended if for no other reason than the hæmostatic effect of well-placed sutures on adjacent vessels. It may also give a more professional, polished appearance to the procedure.

Mr. Hanley points out the necessity of two negative tests to confirm sterility; I certainly agree with this, for, in 63 cases (3·27%) in the group of 1923 vasectomies, a negative test was followed by a positive one. This may explain, or at least illuminate, the case of Mr. D. M. Wallace referred to in the article, in which a single negative test was followed ten months later by positive tests and a pregnant wife. It has also been my observation that, at two months postoperatively, 30% of men had positive tests; at three months, 20%. In view of the rather surprising persistence of sperm in the ejaculate in such a high percentage of men after vasectomy, it may be wise to avoid undue optimism when advising patients as to when contraceptive precautions may be abandoned following the operation. Some men, in my experience, have taken ten or eleven months to obtain two consecutive negative monthly tests (my criterion for success).

I enjoyed reading Mr. Hanley's article, and hope that he will favour us with further details in the light of his continuing experience.

Medical Aspects of Vasectomy

Vasectomy for Contraception

Donald Young

In view of the increasing public interest in vasectomy more surgeons are being approached to perform this operation. As a surgeon who has been working in a male infertility clinic for 20 years I would like to point out some of the pitfalls.

Counsel's opinion for the Medical Defence Union states that the operation is illegal if done only for the purpose of birth control.[1] To cover the surgeon legally it is essential to have a second opinion from a general practitioner, a psychiatrist, or a gynaecologist to the effect that further pregnancies are likely to endanger the mental or physical health of a man's wife.

The surgeon should discuss the operation of bilateral vasectomy, and its implications, with both partners, and obtain the written consent of both husband and wife to the operation.

At operation it is wise to excise 1 cm. from each vas deferens, and both open ends should be ligated with linen thread or silk, rather than catgut. If the excised portions are sent for microscopic examination there can be no doubt that the vas deferens has been tied. Congenital abnormalities of the vas deferens are more common than one thinks.[2] One per cent. of all men attending an infertility clinic have bilateral absence of the vas deferens ; a smaller number have absence of one vas. I have found one case of duplication of the vasa, and probably more will be found as vasectomy becomes more common.

After bilateral ligation of the vas deferens semen analysis must be carried out at monthly intervals for some months to make sure that the seminal reservoir is completely empty of spermatozoa. The patient must be told that contraceptive measures are required until he has had at least one azoospermic ejaculate. If spermatozoa in fair numbers persist for more than three months the possibility of faulty technique, or duplication of the vasa, must be considered and an exploratory operation performed.

REFERENCES

Medical Defence Union Annual Report, 1949.
Wells, C., and Kyle, J., Scientific Foundations of Surgery, 1967, p. 358. London.

Vasectomy for Sterilization

GEORGE WATTS

It seems that, despite the excellent
literature distributed by the Simon Trust,
there are still a number of surgeons who are
not fully conversant with some of the precautions necessary in connexion with this
operation. It is essential that patients have
seminal specimens examined after the operation until two have been obtained which are
free from spermatozoa. In most patients
this is about four to five weeks after the
operation, although others may take several
months. If, however, this has not occurred
at the end of three months then the possibility of the presence of a second vas should
be suspected. This condition, like congenital absence of the vas, is uncommon. It is
obviously of vital importance when a sterilization operation is being performed. If the
patient is examined carefully beforehand it
is possible to palpate the second vas quite
easily, and the operation can still be carried
out through the usual small incisions. I
have also on one occasion seen a patient
where the surgeon had in error ligated the
artery instead of the vas. This should not
occur if the operation is carried out under
proper conditions with adequate lighting in
an operating-theatre. It is unwise for it to
be performed under lesser circumstances.

Another hazard sometimes overlooked is
that patients collect the seminal specimens
from a condom. This is a danger, as the presence of a spermicidal substance may be mis-
leading when examining the fluid, especially
if the specimen had been sent by post and
delayed.

Above all, however, I should like to stress
the importance of making sure that the
patient realizes that it is essential for him to
use normal contraceptive precautions until
azoospermia has been proved.

Men with Vasectomies: A Study of Medical, Sexual, and Psychosocial Changes

ANDREW S. FERBER, M.D., CHRISTOPHER TIETZE, M.D.,
and SARAH LEWIT

Oᴠᴇʀ ᴛʜᴇ ᴘᴀsᴛ few years, the performance of vasectomy has increased in importance as a means of fertility control in the United States and elsewhere. Information obtained in a nationwide survey[1] indicates that about 45,000 such operations are performed annually in the United States. The basic assumption of the present study is that, aside from eliminating the ability to deliver sperm, vasectomy can yield consequences that constitute the psychosocial sequelae of having decided to sterilize oneself. We sought to focus on several questions:

1. How many men and their wives had better, unchanged, and worse outcomes on major sexual, psychological, and social parameters? The self-reports of respondents in prior follow-up studies[2-8] indicate largely favorable outcomes, although a few "bad" outcomes have also been reported.

2. What are the characteristics of those who have "bad" outcomes? Can we develop predictive criteria for subjects who should not have vasectomy? Several detailed post-facto clinical reports in the literature point out instances of sexual pathologic and psychopathologic conditions in men who had undergone vasectomy and attribute the precipitation of symptoms to the operation.[2, 9, 10]

3. What are the typical "trouble spots" before, during, and after the oper-

ation, and how can the physician best assist the patient in coping with them? The trouble spots were: how men decide to have a vasectomy and what doubts make them hesitate, postoperative morbidity, results of sperm tests, typical anxieties surrounding sexual questions, and the possible trauma associated with revealing the operation to others.

We analyzed the data in two ways: (1) description of the demographic characteristics, the medical course, and the sexual, psychological, and sociological outcomes; and (2) correlation between demographic and motivational characteristics (independent variables) and various outcome scores summarizing responses in the areas of physical health, psychosocial adjustment, and sexual satisfaction of husband and wife (as well as coital frequency) as dependent variables. However, no statistically significant correlations were found between the independent variables and outcome scores because of the small numbers of unfavorable outcomes involved.

Method and Materials

Study Outline

The present study is a follow-up of 73 urban-area men who had applied to the Association for Voluntary Sterilization (AVS) for assistance in finding a physician to perform a vasectomy, and who had had the operation in the preceding 5 years.

The interviewers were male residents in psychiatry at medical schools located within the interview areas. A modest honorarium was paid for each completed interview, which lasted about 2 hr. Residents in psychiatry were preferred because it was felt that by training they could exercise greater skill and judgment in obtaining answers to questions of a highly personal and emotional nature.

Letters were sent to the men to be interviewed asking for their cooperation in a study which was "to gather information which will be useful to other men who may consider a vasectomy, to family counselors who give advice on the matter, to physicians who perform the operation, and to hospitals in the formulation of policies." The men were assured that all information would be held in the strictest confidence.

Questionnaire

The questionnaire was developed in collaboration with a number of urologists, psychiatrists, psychologists, and family counselors who were asked to submit lists of questions. The responses were pooled and a draft sent out for critical comments and suggestions. On this basis, a revised draft was tested in the New York City area by one of the authors (A.F.), and further changes made. The final questionnaire, consisting of 96 questions, was divided into 6 segments: personal characteristics, the operation itself, motivational factors, general health, sexual health, and psychosocial adjustment.

Although we believe that the respondents told us how they felt, it should be pointed out that all responses are expressions of the respondent's opinion, bearing a complex and unassessable relationship to his real attitudes. Test-retest reliability was not studied. The questionnaires were coded so that an answer which was only slightly positive was coded as "no change" while even a slight indication of negation was given a negative value. The evaluation of responses and the assigning of code values were the responsibility of the senior author.

Subjects

Primary self-selection and persistent attempts to obtain a vasectomy (often without the help, or even in spite of the disapproval, of their own physicians) characterized the population. This motivational factor may account for the large proportion of favorable results and, also, differentiates the population from the populations studied by Ziegler et al. and others.[2–8, 11, 12]

The 73 men in the study had made their applications to the AVS during the 5-year period from 1956 to 1960, with about three-fourths in the last 2 years of the period. Close to one-half of them lived in the New York City area and the rest were scattered throughout 10 urban areas in the

Northeast, Middle West, and Far West. Rather less than one-half requested financial assistance from the AVS.

In addition to the 73 respondents, 12 men who had received letters refused to be interviewed, of whom 8 filled in a brief questionnaire stating that they were satisfied with the operation but did not wish to be interviewed. Four men failed to respond. This does not appear to be a high ratio of refusals considering the nature of the inquiry and the socioeconomic characteristics of the respondents.

Measured Characteristics

Table 1 shows the distribution of the 73 respondents by various demographic, cultural, and socioeconomic characteristics at time of interview. More than one-half of the men were between 35 and 44, and somewhat more than one-half had been married at least 10 years. None of the respondents was childless, and the great majority had at least 3 children. Most of the men (90%) were white. Somewhat more than one-half of the men stated that they were Protestants, about 1 in 5 was a Roman Catholic, 1 in 10 Jewish, and the remainder was divided between "other faiths" and "no religion."

About one-third of the men had had at least 1 year of college, and one-half possessed high school educations. More men were in professional, managerial, and technical occupations than in any other occupational category; only 2 were in unskilled manual occupations.

A comparison of the socioeconomic characteristics of interviewed men with the same characteristics in the urban population of the United States (according to the 1960 census) reveals two major differences. (1) Men in the professional and managerial occupations were overrepresented among the interviewed group, and those in the semiskilled and unskilled occupations were underrepresented, which points to the subjects' superior economic and educational position. (2) The number of children expected in an urban population of the occupational, ethnic, and age distribution of the interviewed group, according to census data, was about two-thirds of the number observed (2.3 per couple compared with 3.9 per couple), indicating a greater fecundity, or a less successful use of birth control, or both. In general, age differences between husbands and wives tended to be somewhat greater than among urban couples in the census.

TABLE 1. DISTRIBUTION OF DEMOGRAPHIC, CULTURAL, AND SOCIOECONOMIC CHARACTERISTICS

Characteristic	No. of respondents
Total	73
Age	
Less than 35 years	21
35–44 years	39
45 years and older	13
Duration of marriage	
Less than 5 years	9
5–9 years	24
10–14 years	22
15 years and longer	18
No. of children	
1 and 2	10
3 and 4	39
5 and 6	22
7 and more	2
Race	
White	64
Nonwhite	9
Religion	
Protestant	36
Roman Catholic	15
Jewish	8
Other	14
Church attendance	
3 times a month and more	33
Once a month to a few times a year	21
Once a year or less	8
Never	11
Education	
Elementary school: 8 years and less	12
High school: 9–12 years	37
College: 13 years and more	24
Occupation	
Professional, managerial, technical	28
Clerical and sales	9
Skilled manual	17
Semiskilled manual	17
Unskilled manual	2

Motivating Factors

Reasons Stated

One of the questions asked applicants by the AVS is the reason for requesting a vasectomy. One-half (37) of our sample of 73 men stated that they had inadequate economic resources; a slightly smaller number (32) mentioned emotional factors; and a still smaller number (30) offered reasons related to health—either their own or their children's. Seventeen (an average of 4 in 17) stated that they wanted a vasectomy because of previous contraceptive failures. At the time of interview, respondents gave the following answers to the question as to why they changed from other methods of birth control to a permanent one:

Didn't trust other methods	53
Finality of decision	28
Pleasure criteria	22
Anxiety over possible failure	14
Other reasons	1

The number who indicated that they did not trust other methods of contraception (53) exceeded the number who had experienced failures of contraception (48). Of the 73 men in the sample, 71 stated that they had used birth control methods prior to the operation.

Decision Influences

Thirty-eight men had learned about vasectomy through professional channels, family members, or friends, and the remaining 35 through various mass media—particularly through articles published in popular journals (see *Bibliography*). Twelve stated that the operation had been suggested as a "good idea" by professional persons; 11 attributed the suggestion to friends or members of the family. Three felt that they had been *urged* to have the operation.

A majority (43) of those seeking the operation did not discuss it with their physicians, or stated that they had no family doctor. Sixteen were discouraged by their family physicians and sought the operation elsewhere. Only 14 men reported that their family doctors were in favor of the operation.

All 73 men reported that they had discussed the operation with their wives. The responses were:

Agreed	69
Male dominant	9
Female dominant	3
Disagreed	4

"Agreed" means that both parties concurred in the decision; "male dominant" means that the wife complied passively; and "female dominant," that the husband complied passively with the wife's decision. Four women did not agree to the plan and their husbands proceeded unilaterally.

The respondents were asked why they, rather than their wives, had undergone the sterilizing operation. The responses were:

More physical trouble for wife	38
Physician's refusal	16
More family disruption	5
More expensive	5
Other reasons	5
Not considered	15

Forty-eight (2 in 3) respondents had not discussed their plans with friends. Of the 25 men who had, 19 reported an enthusiastic reaction; 3, a neutral reaction; and 3 stated that their friends were opposed.

Twenty-nine men (2 in 5) stated that it took less than 2 weeks for them to decide to have a vasectomy; a somewhat smaller number (24) took more than 2 months; and the remaining 20 men decided in more than 2 weeks but in less than 2 months. Sixteen men had doubts about the operation, which delayed their decision, and 22 were worried or afraid before the operation. Fifty-seven stated that they had had no doubts and 51, that they had not been worried or afraid. The doubts expressed were: (1) the same sort of feeling one would have before any operation; (2) concern about the effects of the operation on their psychosexual status (e.g., "I would feel less of a man," "it might injure my manhood," "it would make me impotent or curb any sexual desire"); (3) projection of fear onto the wife (e.g., "my wife might leave me because I could no longer have kids"); (4) realistic anxieties about a childless future—especially in connection with the possibility of remarriage; and (5) religious scruples.

Further light was thrown on the decision-making process by answers to the question: "Do you feel that you have made a personal sacrifice in having a vasectomy?" Six

101

stated that they had made a personal sacrifice. Some saw it as a sacrifice of a capacity to have children, stressing only the loss to themselves. Others emphasized the sacrifice for someone else—the wife or the whole family.

Results

Medical Aspects

Fifty-nine of the 73 operations were performed in a physician's office, and 14 in a hospital, among which 6 patients required 1 day of hospitalization, and 8, 2 or more days. A majority of the men (40) did not spend any days at home after the operation; 9 stayed home for 1 day; and 24, for 2 or more days. Local anesthesia was used in 65 cases, and general anesthesia in 8.

No pain during the operation was experienced by 52 men, while 21 reported pain. Severe complications following the operation were reported in 3 cases: 2 ambulatory wound infections and 1 bilateral scrotal hematoma that became infected and required drainage, with the patient hospitalized. In addition, 15 men reported minor complications (e.g., swelling of the testicles), most of which lasted for 2 weeks or less. The men were asked to give their subjective estimate of the discomfort experienced during the operation, compared with anticipated discomfort. Thirty-four reported the operation was "as anticipated," 21 found it less unpleasant, and 18, more unpleasant than expected.

Success in Preventing Pregnancy

In 70 of the 73 cases, no postoperative pregnancy occurred, while in 3 cases, pregnancy had occurred. These 3 failures illustrate the need on the part of the physician to make the patient aware that postoperative sperm tests must be made.

In one case of reported failure, the wife became pregnant 14 months after the operation. The man had not had any sperm tests because he "thought the operation was successful" and he "was probably too lazy." He also failed to return for treatment of a wound infection in the immediate postoperative period, again because of "laziness." In another failure, pregnancy occurred 3 months after the operation. The man had had his last sperm test 1 month after the vasectomy. A subsequent vasectomy proved successful. The third case of failure involves a man who continued to have positive sperm counts after two vasectomies. This man is now using condoms and is, understandably enough, disillusioned about the vasectomy procedure.

Postoperative Sperm Tests

In spite of the importance of postoperative sperm tests, 13 men reported that they did not have any, and 19 reported their last test had been made less than 1 month after the operation. In 18 additional cases, sperm tests were made 1–2 months after the operation, and in 22 cases, 2 months and more after operation. Only 1 sperm test had been made in 33 cases, and 2 or more, in 26. For 1 man, no information on sperm tests was available.

The reasons given by the 13 men for not having sperm tests were: not being told about them, laziness, and embarrassment at having to masturbate (which can easily be avoided by the use of condom specimens obtained during coitus).

Resumption of Sexual Activity

The time interval between the operation and the resumption of sexual activity was as follows:

4 weeks and more	30
2–4 weeks	25
1–2 weeks	13
3–7 days	4
Less than 3 days	1

Fifteen men reported transient discomfort on one or more occasions during intercourse; all but 2 ceased within 3 months. The 2 men reported a tenderness in the testicles for 6–12 months during vigorous intercourse.

Outcome Parameters

The outcome questions on the questionnaire almost all took the form of asking each respondent to compare his own or his wife's condition, behavior, or attitude at the time of the interview with the same variables retrospectively. Thus, each respondent served as his own control and set his own base line.

The areas chosen for investigation for possible change were: (1) physical health; (2) sexual behavior; (3) psychosocial adjustment factors—including marital, job, and community relationships and concern about children; (4) satisfaction with the operation; and (5) social behavior with regard to the operation.

Physical Health

Most of the respondents (68) stated that their health was excellent or good, and only 5 judged their health as being "fair" (Table 2). "Fair" health was assigned to a somewhat larger proportion of wives (14); 1 husband reported his wife in poor health. Compared with their health prior to the operation, 11

TABLE 2. HUSBAND'S REPORT OF OWN AND WIFE'S PRE- AND POSTOPERATIVE HEALTH STATUS

	Husband	Wife
HEALTH AT TIME OF INTERVIEW		
Excellent	40	20
Good	28	38
Fair	5	14
Poor	—	1
COMPARED WITH PREOPERATIVE HEALTH		
Better	6	22
Same	62	50
Worse	5	1

men reported changes for themselves, and 23 men for their wives. Of the 11 men who reported changes in health, 6 felt that the changes were for the better and 5, for the worse. The respondents felt that their wives' health had improved in 22 cases and had worsened in 1 case.

Few of the men felt that any changes in their own health were attributable to the operation. Two of the 6 in better health and 1 of the 5 in worse health attributed the changes to the operation. On the other hand, 13 of the 22 men who reported an improvement in the health of their wives felt that the change was related to the operation. Many of the improvements referred to mental health, e.g., "my wife doesn't worry herself crazy before her periods anymore," and "she no longer has anemia and fatigue from all the babies in so few years."

The psychiatrist-interviewers' estimates of the general level of psychopathology referred more to character and to chronic aspects than to acute anxiety or depression at the time of the interview. These estimates can be summed up as follows:

Severe psychopathology	4
Moderate psychopathology	32
Well-integrated	37

This distribution approximates estimates of mental health found in samples of the general population.[13] Four men had a history of prior psychiatric treatment; 1 had treatment after the operation and 1 had treatment both before and after it. However, no systematic correlation could be demonstrated between psychiatric status at the time of interview and outcome on sexual and other parameters.

A summary of postvasectomy changes in "physical" habits such as, smoking, appetite, etc., included in the study appears in Table 3. Weight changes (5 lb. or more) were reported as follows: more, 13; same, 56; less, 4; no change, 0.

The data on health seem to indicate an average population which changed

TABLE 3. Habit Changes after Vasectomy

Parameter	Use or degree			
	More	Same	Less	No change
Sleep	4	69	0	0
Smoking	5	42	4	22
Alcohol	2	49	4	18
Appetite	3	67	3	0
Exercise	10	49	4	10

little and randomly after vasectomy. The improvement in the health of the wives is worthy of comment. It runs a gamut from decreased premenstrual anxiety, through the psychosomatic borderlands of less fatigue and lethargy, to improvement in varicose veins, all of which seem clearly attributable to not being pregnant frequently. No support was found for the notion that a wife may fall sick as a conversion phenomenon after the sterilization of her husband. Of the 5 men who reported a setback in their health, 1 developed Hodgkin's disease within a year of his vasectomy and was preoccupied with the possibility of some connection between the two. The others saw no connections between the operation and any deterioration in health. The validity of these data is limited by the fact that single interviews cannot reveal unconscious conflicts.

Sexual Behavior

Because of the frequent concern of patients and physicians with the effect of vasectomy on sexual behavior, this area was scrutinized and analyzed with particular care. Data are reported for individual items, and two scales were constructed for male and female satisfaction and were correlated with independent variables.

COITAL FREQUENCY. Although the men were on the average 4 years older at the time of the interview than they had been at the time of the vasectomy, the mean coital frequency increased from 8.4 to 9.8 times per month, and the median changed from 10.3 to 12.6 times per month. On the basis of data reported by Kinsey and his associates, a decline of 1.2 in mean monthly coital frequency might have been expected in this age interval.[14]

MALE SEXUAL SATISFACTION. Somewhat more than two-thirds of the men (50) stated that they felt freer and less inhibited sexually than before the operation, and somewhat less than one-third (22) reported no change (Table 4). One stated that he felt less free. According to the men's self-rating of "over-all satisfaction with coitus" after the operation, three-fourths (55) were more satisfied, and one-fifth (15) reported no change. Three men stated that they were less satisfied.

The self-ratings on duration of ejaculation and quality of orgasm, and on control over ejaculation were similar, with about three-fifths of the men reporting no change, between one-fifth

TABLE 4. Husband's Report on Changes in Own Sexual Satisfaction

Factor	Much more	Little more	No change	Little less
Feeling of freedom and decreased inhibition	10	40	22	1
Satisfaction with coitus	6	49	15	3
Duration of ejaculation and strength of orgasm	4	10	45	14*
Control over ejaculation	1	17	46	9
Ease and strength of erection	2	6	58	7†

*Includes 1 man who reported much shorter and weaker ejaculation and orgasm.
†Includes 1 man who reported much more difficult and weaker erections.

104

and one-fourth reporting improvement, and the remainder (between one-fifth and one-tenth) reporting deterioration. With regard to the men's self-evaluation of the quality and ease of erection, four-fifths of the men stated that no change had occurred, while almost equal numbers of the remainder (8 and 7, respectively) reported either an improvement or a worsening in the quality and ease of erection.

FEMALE SEXUAL SATISFACTION. Since the interviews were conducted with the husbands, only the husbands' evaluation of their wives' sexual satisfaction, which may or may not differ from their wives' own evaluation, can be presented here. Three different criteria were used as measures of sexual satisfaction.

1. Close to four-fifths of the husbands (57) reported that their wives felt less inhibited and freer sexually, one-fifth (15) were unchanged, and 1 wife was reported as being more inhibited (Table 5).

2. Thirty-six men reported that their wives reached climax more easily, 35 reported no change, and 2 men reported a lessened ability to reach climax on the part of their wives.

3. Close to two-fifths of the wives (29) were reported by their husbands as initiating love play leading to coitus more often than before the operation, somewhat less than three-fifths (42) as not having changed, and 2 as initiating love play less often.

According to their husbands, most women who improved on any one item improved on either or both of the other two items, and none of them decreased her satisfaction on any other item. A distribution of individual responses shows that only 9 women were reported by their husbands as experiencing no change on all three items. Three women were reported by their husbands as having decreased their satisfaction on one or more items and none of the 3 showed improvement on any item. Three men and 3 women were less satisfied with their sex lives after the operation, according to the respondents' statements.

OTHER TYPES OF SEXUAL BEHAVIOR. The men were asked questions on other types of sexual behavior, such as nocturnal emissions, daydreams, masturbation, extramarital coitus, homosexual activities, and whether they experienced fantasies about their genitalia being mutilated or cut off. Because of the infrequency and the variable nature of both the phenomena and their perceptibility, the responses did not lend themselves to quantitative analysis. They are discussed here because questions on these subjects are often raised in considering the outcome of vasectomy operations.

We were especially interested in the question on extramarital coitus because of the widely circulated rumor that men who are sterilized become promiscuous. Only one man reported increased extramarital coitus. He had been having an affair before the vasectomy and was less fearful about it afterward. Responses to this question from other men were: "Just after the operation I thought I would be a big Don Juan, but that passed away soon and I'm faithful to my wife." "I think less about other women than I did, I guess it's because I'm more satisfied now." "I have fewer

TABLE 5. HUSBAND'S REPORT ON CHANGES IN WIFE'S SEXUAL SATISFACTION

Factor	Much more	Little more	No change	Little less
Feeling of freedom and decreased inhibition	13	44	15	1
Ability to reach climax	8	28	35	2
Initiation of love play	5	24	42	2

fantasies about other women." "I used to have frequent fantasies and some affairs before the vasectomy, but none since. Probably because my wife seems to have changed."

One man reported an increase in masturbation, inexplicable to himself. Ideas, dreams, or thoughts that connote or mention genital mutilation were reported by several men. As outlined below under *Social Behavior,* it is our belief that such ideas must occur in all men undergoing the procedure.

Psychosocial

More men noted improvements in their wives' tension levels than in their own. Two-thirds of the wives (49) were reported by their husbands as being less tense compared with only two-fifths of the husbands (31). More than one-half of the men (40) reported no change in their own tension levels, while one-fourth (19) reported no change for their wives. Greater tension was reported for 2 husbands and for 5 wives.

Forty-six men (about 2 in 3) reported that they considered their relations with their wives prior to the operation better than most. Ten men felt that, prior to the operation, they did not get along with their wives as well as might be desired. All but 2 of the men questioned felt that this relationship had either remained the same or improved.

Most men reported no postoperative change in their ability to get along with their fellow workers (67), in their work enjoyment (65), and in their feelings of job security (63). Improvement in all three of these sectors was reported by 6, 6, and 7 men, respectively. Two men reported decreased enjoyment of their work, and 3 men, a lessening of their feeling of job security.

Fifty-three reported an increase in their feelings of over-all happiness, emphasizing such factors as peace, stability, decision-making, and the possibility of planning for the future. Two men reported themselves as less happy. The

remaining 18 men experienced no change in their self-assessment of their own happiness.

Sixty-five of the respondents stated that the operation had not increased their concern over their children, while 8 reported that it had.

Postoperation Attitudes

Satisfaction

In spite of the variety of responses on various factors, 72 of the 73 men stated that, given the chance, they would have the operation again. The only man who said that he would not do so had already undergone 2 unsuccessful operations. Of the 73 men, 71 stated that they would recommend the operation to others. The 2 negative responses came from men who feared to make a recommendation because then "they would know I have had one."

Social Behavior

In spite of the statement of most respondents that they would recommend the operation, only 35 had actually done so. An examination of the responses to the question regarding whether the respondent cared whether other people knew that he had undergone a vasectomy revealed that one-half (36) did and one-half (37) did not. Forty-eight men had told members of their family and their friends that they had been operated on, and 25 had not told anyone. Among the reasons given for not wanting others to know were: "what they would say; they are Catholics" (15); "because it's none of their business" (19); and shame (4).

The inquiry was an especially *charged* one. Some interviewers observed that many subjects flinched and showed tension when asked—even those who said they didn't care. It seemed clear that most men assumed a loss of status attendant upon sterilization, and while willing to deal with their own internal self-critique, were reluctant to face the

106

disapproval of others. Some of the reported reactions of persons told about the vasectomy were: "People think it's a form of castration and affects potency." "My brother-in-law thought it unmanly. My Catholic friends said 'How could you?'" "My brother said, 'If I had one, I'd turn into a fairy. In a few years, I wouldn't have any organs left.'" "My friends are generally interested and think it's a good idea."

Some of the reasons advanced by the respondents for not telling others about their vasectomy were: "Some men will fear change in sex life." "People have prejudices. Would influence their opinion of my masculinity in some way." "People will make fun of you." "I'm a Catholic. They'd think I was bad." "In-laws would blame my wife for forcing me into it." "My wife thinks others would want affairs with me if they knew."

These responses seem to highlight several points. We feel vasectomy does stimulate infantile fears and fantasies of castration, impotence, and concomitant decline in self-esteem. Many responses about telling people seem to be externalizations onto a vague "other" of a man's negative feelings about himself having had the operation. Most of these men, we feel, successfully cope with these fantasies stimulated by the operation and do not develop overt psychosexual pathology. However, some men fail to cope with their fantasies, and present cases where psychosexual difficulties are traced to and blamed on vasectomy. From a different angle, the social stigma attached to this operation is still quite high. It stimulates fantasies in others, such as the ones respondents report hearing from people they have told about the matter.

It appears to us that many difficulties could be avoided by widely circulating, in popular and medical literature, the known results of vasectomy to allay the fears of both physicians and the general public; by stressing strict confidentiality in all professional dealings with men seeking or undergoing vasectomy; and by warning the men of the possibility of others having critical attitudes towards them, suggesting that they be circumspect in talking about the operation. Such advice from a physician can help the men cope with the required psychological adjustments.

Discussion

The findings of general improvement on sexual and psychosocial parameters after vasectomy parallel those of several other postoperative interviews and questionnaire surveys.[2-8] The especially positive results our respondents report may have to do with the high motivation of our sample in seeking this operation.

What is the relationship of sexual and psychosocial pathology to an antecedent vasectomy, and how high are the chances that difficulties will occur? Two published reports that emphasize this relationship are those of Erickson[9] and Johnson.[10] Erickson's 6 cases are gathered from his psychotherapeutic practice. He describes men who chose the operation for clearly symbolic and self-mutilative reasons. Johnson's sample of men was drawn from those already admitted to a VA psychiatric hospital.

We agree with some of the conclusions of these authors: that vasectomy is perceived by all men, on some level, in some way, as a castration. We believe this attitude is supported by our data on reactions of friends and relatives told about the operation, reasons given by respondents for not telling, worries before the operation, and the heightened defensiveness shown by respondents when being questioned about the meaning of the operation.

We differ on the following crucial point: the relative psychopathogenicity of the operation as such. We consider mastering the psychodynamic factors of

"I will be sterile, castrated, no good," as one of the tasks a man must go through during adjustment to a vasectomy. The changed self-image is only one of several interacting psychological and social motives, including the sense of mastery and relief at having taken one's destiny into one's hands; the achieved control of a fertility that was becoming more a curse than a blessing; the loss of fear of further pregnancies, etc. Our data indicate that the overwhelming majority of our respondents have been able to cope with the general task adequately, and report an over-all higher level of satisfaction with life. Johnson's and Erickson's cases came from groups already psychologically decompensated.

Who demonstrated "bad" or equivocal outcomes, and what can a study of their cases tell us about indications for denying a request for voluntary sterilization? Three men stated that they felt less satisfied with their sexual lives after the operation. Each had a pre-existing potency difficulty that was aggravated after the operation. One reported his wife much more satisfied with their mutual sex life after the operation; the second felt there had been no change; and the third had the only wife who was reported by her husband as much "worse" in her sexual expression.

Our clinical impressions were that the strongest contraindication for vasectomy is disagreement with one's wife over its advisability. Only 4 of our men had disagreed with their wives. Two of these showed our 2 worst results in terms of sexual behavior. A third was a man who, while stating his sexual life was the same, gave evidence of increased chronic neurotic tension and worry, and whose wife still held his lack of trust in her against him. The fourth subject in this group was a man whose sex life was more bound up with his mistress than with his wife. We infer that sterilization as an attempt to salvage a failing marriage seems to carry a bad prognosis.

Still another contraindication mentioned in literature is an admitted assent to the operation on the basis of another's urging. However, of the 3 cases of this type in our study, only 1 subject was rated as a bad male sexual outcome and the other 2 reported increased sexual satisfaction and increased happiness. It is therefore proposed that the effects of "being urged" be further investigated. Along the same line, the possibility of a poor outcome among men seeing the operation as a personal sacrifice was also investigated. Of the 6 men who reported such feelings, all 6 reported increased sexual satisfaction, and 5 of the 6, better psychosocial adjustments.

Of the 5 men with a history of prior psychiatric treatment, none had equivocal or "bad" outcomes on any parameter. Four men who showed sufficient psychopathology at interview to be diagnosed as showing severe psychopathology reported increased sexual satisfaction for themselves and their wives and improved psychosocial adjustment. We also conclude that religion, education, number of children, history of psychiatric treatment, and psychotic symptoms per se do *not* carry a poor psychosocial prognosis.

Serious reservations are raised as to the meaning of our data by Rodgers et al.,[11, 12] who studied couples who had sought vasectomy voluntarily. Their design was a longitudinal one with pre-operative and 1-year postoperative use of questionnaires, interviews, and Minnesota Multiphasic Personality Inventories (MMPI). These investigators' questionnaire and interview data are parallel to ours on all major parameters (sexual behavior and satisfaction, marital happiness, work, health, lack of extramarital affairs). On the MMPI there were significant changes that indicated increased psychological disturbance in a significant portion of their tested subjects. We cannot compare our data to theirs because we used neither a longitudinal design nor objective measures.

Summary

A total of 73 men who had applied for a vasectomy to the AVS and who were interviewed 1 to 5 years after the operation, reported as follows:

1. Seventy anatomically successful operations and 3 failures.

2. No change in their own physical health, and a slight tendency toward improvement in the health of their wives.

3. A significant increase in coital frequency at an age when the frequency for the general population is declining.

4. Fifty-five (3 of 4) men more satisfied with intercourse, 15 no change, and 3 less satisfied.

5. Sixty-one wives reported by husbands as more satisfied with sexual intercourse, 9 no change, and 3 less satisfied.

6. Improvement on psychosocial parameters of self and wife's tension levels, relations with wife, and over-all happiness were reported by between one-fourth and one-half of the husbands. Most of the rest, unchanged; some deterioration on each of these parameters reported by from 2 to 5 men. Work relationships remained unaffected.

7. Seventy-two men would make the same decision again; the 1 dissenter had had two operative failures.

8. Disagreement with wife over the desirability of sterilization seemed to favor development of later psychosocial pathology.

9. Evidence is presented that these men and their friends and relatives hold stereotyped attitudes equating vasectomy with being castrated and made inferior, and that the good results indicate adequate coping with these psychological factors by a large majority of the respondents.

References

1. CAMPBELL, A. A. The incidence of operations that prevent conception. *Amer J Obstet Gynec* 89:694, 1964.

2. DANDEKAR, K. After-effects of vasectomy. *Artha Vijnana* (Gokhale Institute of Politics and Economics, Poona, India) 5:212, 1963.

3. GARRISON, P. L., and GAMBLE, C. J. Sexual effects of vasectomy. *JAMA* 144:293, 1950.

4. LANDIS, J. T., and POFFENBERGER, T. The marital and sexual adjustment of 330 couples who chose vasectomy as a form of birth control. *J Marriage and the Family* 27:57, 1965.

5. PHADKE, G. M. Vasectomy. *J Indian Med Ass* 37:241, 1961.

6. POFFENBERGER, S. B., and SHETH, D. L. Reactions of urban employees to vasectomy operations. *J Family Welfare* 10:7, 1963.

7. POFFENBERGER, T., and POFFENBERGER, S. B. Vasectomy as a preferred method of birth control: A preliminary investigation. *Marriage and Family Living* 25:326, 1963.

8. ZIEGLER, F. J., RODGERS, D. A., and KRIEGSMAN, S. A. Effect of vasectomy on psychological functioning. Paper presented at the Annual Meeting of the American Psychosomatic Society, Philadelphia, May 1965.

9. ERICKSON, M. H. "The Psychological Significance of Vasectomy." In *Therapeutic Abortion*. H. Rosen, Ed. Julian Press, New York, 1954.

10. JOHNSON, M. H. Social and psychological effects of vasectomy. *Amer J Psychiat* 121:482, 1964.

11. RODGERS, D. A., ZIEGLER, F. J., ROHR, P., and PRENTISS, R. J. Sociopsychological characteristics of patients obtaining vasectomies from urologists. *Marriage and Family Living* 25:331, 1963.

12. RODGERS, D. A., ZIEGLER, F. J., ALTROCCHI, J., and LEVY, N. A longitudinal study of the psycho-social effects of vasectomy. *J Marriage and the Family* 27:59, 1965.

13. SROLE, L., LANGNER, T. S., MICHAEL, S. T., OPLER, M., and RENNIE, T. A. C.

Mental Health in the Metropolis: the Midtown Manhattan Study. McGraw-Hill, New York, 1962, p. 216.

14. KINSEY, A. C., POMEROY, W. B., and MARTIN, C. E. *Sexual Behavior in the Human Male.* Saunders, Philadelphia, 1948, Table 56, p. 252.

Bibliography

STOKES, W. R. Long-range effects of male sterilization. *Sexology* Oct. 1965; GOODMAN, W. Abortion and sterilization. *Redbook* Oct. 1965; Surgery-voluntary sterilization. *Time* Jan. 15, 1965; RIDGEWAY, J. Birth control by surgery. *New Republic* Nov. 14, 1964; BRENTON M. The most controversial method of birth control. *Coronet* July 1964; Anonymous. The operation that stops pregnancy. *Real Romances* June 1964; GUTTMACHER, A. F. Facts and arguments—sterilization. *The Nation* Apr. 6, 1964; LAIDLOW, R. W. Birth control. *N Y Herald Tribune* Feb. 15, 1964; RAGUE, J. R. Voluntary sterilization. *Med World News* Dec. 20, 1963; The male operation. *Newsweek* Sept. 16, 1963; GUTTMACHER, A. F. I just can't face having another baby. *True Story* Nov. 1959.

LACATE DEHYDROGENASE ISOZYME PATTERNS IN PRE- AND POSTVASECTOMY SEMINAL PLASMA

K. H. Moon and R. G. Bunge

Lactate dehydrogenase (LDH), an enzyme of the glycolytic cycle, has been found in all tissues and in body fluids with glycolytic activity. LDH isozyme consists of five heterogenous isozymes and has been applied in the diagnosis of different diseases (1, 2). It was found, however, that there are six isozymes in human spermatozoa and seminal plasma and in extracts of mature testes from different mammalian species and this extra band originated from spermatozoa (3–7). LDH isozyme patterns were recorded in this laboratory by fluorometric scanning method and their interpretation was attempted. This paper presents the results of LDH isozyme patterns of pre- and postvasectomy seminal plasma to elucidate the LDH patterns in normal fertile seminal plasma.

MATERIALS AND METHODS

Pre- and postvasectomy semen samples were obtained from 12 fertile males. Prevasectomy semen samples were obtained and postvasectomy samples were obtained from the same subjects four weeks after surgery. All of the prevasectomy semen samples had normal semenograms with known fertile capability and postvasectomy semens were azoospermic. Semen samples were centrifuged within 30 min after collection and the supernatants were used for this study. One microliter of seminal plasma was loaded in the well of Agarose Universal Electrophoresis film and the separation of LDH isozyme was obtained by the Turner's Electrophoresis Cell (Turner model 310) and detected through a Turner's Fluorometer and recorded on a Bausch and Lomb recorder (8). Also the migrating patterns in Agarose strips were observed under ultraviolet light. Although the migrating patterns were constantly reproduced

This study was supported by Grant M66.075 from the Population Council, Incorporated, Rockefeller Institute, New York, New York.

by this method, the quantitation of LDH isozyme was not reproducible in the semen sample. Quantitative assays were therefore not attempted.

The essential differences in the migrating patterns of LDH isozymes in pre- and postvasectomy seminal plasma in 12 subjects were similar; only three subjects were selected to present the LDH patterns in pre- and post-vasectomy seminal plasma in Figure 1. The LDH isozyme patterns in pre-vasectomy seminal plasma showed invariably six components and this extra component (LDHx) was located between LDH 3 and 4. LDH 1 is the leading anodal band. As demonstrated in Figure 1, the extra component (LDHx) is not completely separated from LDH 3 and 4 because this band fills gaps between LDH 3 and 4 bands. It was, however, clearly demonstrated by ultra-violet light that the extra band (LDHx) was completely separated from LDH 3 and 4. It was not possible to photograph the fluorescent bands in the Agarose strip; therefore, schematic representation of each band is placed at the base of each isozyme pattern for ease of comparison. The LDH patterns in postvasectomy seminal plasma showed only five components and an extra band (LDHx) seen in prevasectomy seminal plasma was completely absent.

DISCUSSION

All of the prevasectomy seminal plasmas of known fertile subjects have shown a unique extra band (LDHx) between 3 and 4 and this extra band disappeared after vasectomy. Since postvasectomy seminal plasma is constituted mainly by seminal and prostatic secretion, the extra band could be of testicular origin. Furthermore, another study showed there was no extra band in tissue extracts of the epididymis, the vas deferens, the prostate gland, the immature testicular tissue, or the azoospermic seminal fluid. On the contrary, mature testicular tissue, normospermic and oligospermic seminal plasma showed six components. From this experimental study it is obvious that the extra band originated specifically from spermatozoa and this molecular form of LDHx probably reflects a very specific metabolic requirement of spermatozoa. The presence of LDHx in seminal plasma, the whole ejaculate, and washed spermatozoa probably indicates that this specific isozyme had already been secreted from spermatozoa before ejaculation or from dead or injured spermatozoa during centrifugation. As we mentioned before, it was not possible to quantitate each component of isozyme by these methods; however, it was presumed that there might be certain quantitative correlation between LDHx and the number, activity, and viability of spermatozoa. It is therefore suggested that quantitative assay of LDHx in seminal plasma, in seminal fluid, or spermatozoa could lead to a method to elucidate the metabolic activity of spermatozoa and might be applicable to some aspects of male infertility.

Acknowledgment. The authors gratefully acknowledge the technical help of Charles Kingsbury.

112

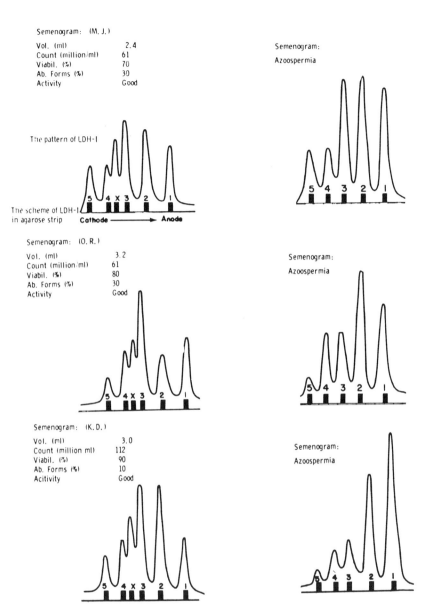

FIG. 1. LDH isozyme patterns in prevasectomy (*left*) and postvasectomy (*right*) seminal plasmas.

REFERENCES

1. Vessell, D. S., and Bearn, A. G.: Isoenzymes of lactic dehydrogenase in human tissues. J. Clin. Invest., *40:* 586, 1961.
2. Wroblewski, F., and Gregory, K. F.: Lactic dehydrogenase isoenzymes and their

distribution in normal tissues and plasma and in disease states. Ann. N.Y. Acad. Sci., *94:* 912, 1961.

3. Zinkham, W. H., Blanco, A., and Kupchyk, L.: Lactate dehydrogenase in testis: Dissociation and recombination of subunits. Science, *142:* 1303, 1963.

4. Blanco, A., and Zinkham, W. H.: Lactate dehydrogenases in human testes. Science, *139:* 601, 1963.

5. Goldberg, E.: Lactic and malic dehydrogenases in human spermatozoa. Science, *139:* 602, 1963.

6. Clausen, J., and Øvlisen, B.: Lactate dehydrogenase isoenzymes of human semen. Biochem. J., *97:* 513, 1965.

7. Elevitch, F. R., and Phillips, R. E.: Lactate dehydrogenase in serum: Estimation by the kinetic fluorometric method. A clinical laboratory procedure from G. K. Turner Associates, Inc., Palo Alto, California, March 1966.

8. Zinkham, W. H., Blanco, A., and Clowry, L. J.: An unusual isozyme of lactate dehydrogenase in mature testes: Localization, ontogeny and kinetic properties. Ann. N.Y. Acad. Sci., *121:* 571, 1964.

Sperm-agglutinating Autoantibodies in Relation to Male Infertility

Dr Ph Rümke

It is now well established that some infertile human males possess autoantibodies against spermatozoa. As was originally described by Wilson (1954), these autoantibodies agglutinate and sometimes immobilize the otherwise normal spermatozoa in the ejaculate. The agglutinated spermatozoa can no longer penetrate the cervical mucus, so that the patient is infertile.

Sperm agglutinins are present in seminal fluid as well as in blood plasma and they are specific for spermatozoa (Rümke 1954, Rümke & Hellinga 1959). Variation exists in the agglutination type. Most sera agglutinate the spermatozoa by their tails or by tails and heads, while some sera only agglutinate the heads. In general there is a parallel between serum titres and the inability of the patients' spermatozoa to invade the cervical mucus (Rümke & Hellinga 1959, Fjällbrant 1965). However, there are exceptions to this rule: some patients have strong autoagglutination with rather low serum titres, and occasionally a patient has only partial and slow-starting agglutination in spite of a high serum titre (Rümke & Hellinga 1959).

A macroscopical agglutination technique with normal sperm of various donors, as designed by Kibrick et al. (1952), was used by us to examine serum samples routinely (Rümke & Hellinga 1959). Out of 2,015 infertile males only 67 patients ($3 \cdot 3\%$) were found with titres of 1:32 or higher, whereas the serum of 416 fertile males and 124 unselected infertile women never possessed

115

sperm agglutinins at that titre. Semen analysis showed a normal sperm density and initial motility in about one-third of these 67 patients, in whom autoagglutination was usually also present. Another third had oligospermia, often with subnormal motility, in which group auto-agglutination was not often easy to observe. The remaining third consisted of patients with azoospermia, which was nearly always due to obstruction of the efferent ducts. Testis biopsies performed in 17 cases of azoospermia revealed normal histology in 15 instances and only partial abnormalities in 2 cases. Thus, just as in animal experiments, sperm autoantibodies are not capable of interfering with spermatogenesis.

The finding of sperm agglutinins in the serum of patients with obstructed efferent ducts has also been reported by others. Phadke & Padukone (1964) found sperm agglutinins in the serum of 8 out of 25 men whose vasa had been ligated as a family limitation measure two to twenty years previously. Recently we tested the serum of 11 patients with congenital absence of both vasa deferentia and seminal vesicles, and in 5 of the 11 we found sperm agglutinins (titres: 1:8, 1:16, 1:16, 1:32, 1:256) (Rümke & Kremer 1967, unpublished). In cases of obstruction many pathologists have observed extravasation of sperm into the interstitium of the epididymis accompanied by infiltration of mononuclears, and even spermatozoa in the lymph vessels (see Rümke 1965). Numerous animal experiments, some performed as early as the turn of the century, have shown that spermatozoa or testicular substances can evoke autoantibodies to spermatozoa (see Rümke 1965) and in man it has been demonstrated by Mancini et al. (1965) that patients with prostatic carcinoma immunized with their own testicular tissue incorporated in complete Freund's adjuvant develop antibodies specifically reacting with spermatozoa. Thus patients who resorb their own spermatozoa may be expected to respond with autoantibody formation against spermatozoa.

One can ask why three-quarters of the males with obstruction do not develop sperm agglutinins in spite of presumed excessive resorption. Phadke (1964) has not regularly observed sperm extravasation in the epididymis in such cases, and a variable mechanism of sperm phagocytosis could account for differences in autoantibody response. Extraneous material is resorbed by phagocytosis and intracellular digestion in various cells lining the sperm pathway. Burgos (1967) suggests that a defective digestive process could allow the escape of incompletely digested and so potentially antigenic molecules. Sperm digestion may be disturbed by spermiostasis, trauma or inflammation. Other possible explanations for the variable sperm agglutination formation in cases of obstruc-

Table 1
Serum of patients with congenital absence of vasa deferentia

Case	Age (years)	Sperm agglutinin titres	γG	γA	γM	Anti-measles CF titres
			(% of standard serum)			
VW	32	256	104	87	85	64
JW	37	32	120	91	150	16
LH	38	16	114	111	?	16
CT	31	16	75	76	64	32
JV	34	8	90	89	111	64
JD	32	—	64	46	114	8
HD	44	—	85	69	49	8
AM	35	—	79	40	52	—
CP	26	—	79	54	102	8
HT	40	—	116	69	80	—
WW	33	—	96	53	88	16
				$P = 0.004$		$P = 0.008$

tion are: (1) Resorption of sperm antigens may also induce immune tolerance. (2) An 'adjuvant' inflammatory effect may be necessary to initiate antibody formation. (3) Other kinds of antibodies could block the formation of agglutinating antibodies. (4) Weakly antigenic stimuli may be effective only with individuals genetically more prone to produce antibodies than others.

The last consideration can be sustained by the following observation: The sera of the 11 above-mentioned patients with congenital absence of the vasa deferentia were examined for the concentration of gamma G, A and M and for the titre of complement-fixing antibodies to measles virus. The patients with sperm agglutinins all had higher levels of gamma A in their serum than those without sperm agglutinins (Table 1). Further, the titres of anti-measles virus antibodies were also higher in the group with the sperm agglutinins.

That obstruction might lead to excessive resorption and so to antibody formation is also suggested by studying our non-azoospermic patients. Among these, case histories and physical examination often indicated the likelihood of obstruction on one side (Rümke 1965); they either had healed gonorrhœal or tuberculous epididymitis or had undergone a herniorrhaphy in childhood (during this operation an inexperienced surgeon may cut the tiny vasa deferentia). One of our patients had developed an acute necrosis of one testis after a surgical accident during herniorrhaphy in adult life. However, in more than half of these patients no cause for autoantibody formation was found. Moreover, in 3, surgical exploration found no evidence of obstruction in epididymis and vas deferens. Whether in such cases the sperm is resorbed in the testis itself or in the rete testis remains thus far an open question.

Another possible explanation for the sperm agglutinin formation is suggested from the experimental work of Weil and his co-workers (see Weil 1965). These authors found that spermatozoa receive a coating of an antigen derived from the

116

seminal vesicles when they become admixed to the combined secretions of the adnexal glands. Since it was believed that the substance was organ-specific it could be postulated that an autoimmune syndrome of the vesicles might exist and that in this case autoantibodies against the coating-antigen would manifest themselves as sperm agglutinins. However, Hekman & Rümke (1967, unpublished) could identify a potent coating antigen originating from the vesicles as lacto-ferrin. Lactoferrin had already been found by Masson & Heremans (1966) to be a common antigen of milk and seminal plasma and other body fluids. Since it does not seem very likely that such a non-organ-specific protein as lactoferrin would ever induce autoantibodies, it is unlikely that sperm agglutinins would primarily be directed to this coating antigen.

If the autoantibody formation is the result of sperm resorption then the sperm antibodies should react with testicular spermatozoa. We therefore examined our sperm-agglutinating patients' sera with the indirect immunofluores-cent antibody technique for their capacity to stain ejaculated spermatozoa as compared with spermatozoa in testicular cryostat sections. The preliminary results (Feltkamp *et al.* 1965) revealed that most of the stronger agglutinating sera stained parts of the heads or the midpieces of the ejaculated spermatozoa. A few non-agglutina-ting sera stained heads; nevertheless a positive correlation was found between agglutination and fluorescent staining. The correlation of the stained sperm part and agglutination type, how-ever, was not clear. Tail staining was considered to be an artifact. Spermatozoa in testicular sections were often stained with the sera that also stained the ejaculated spermatozoa, indicating that in these instances the antibodies were reacting with an antigen of testicular origin. Some sera appeared to react either with ejaculated or with testicular spermatozoa only. The results of experiments recently performed (Hamerlynck & Rümke 1967, unpublished) with 11 sera that agglutinated spermatozoa in dilutions of 1:512 or higher and with non-agglutinating sera are sum-marized in Table 2; 8 of the 11 agglutinating sera stained either sperm heads or midpieces. When the air-dried sperm smears were fixed with metha-nol the staining of the heads was more clearly

Table 2
Fluorescent staining of sperm heads or midpieces

Sera	Total	−	⊥	+ <1:10	+ + ≥1:10
Sperm-agglutinating (1:512), infertile patients	11	1	0	2	8
Non-agglutinating, men over 67	88	42	16	22	8
				P<0·002	

visible and seemed more specific, abolishing most staining in controls and any staining of the mid-pieces. Some of the non-agglutinating sera, obtained from males whose age was more than 67 years, weakly stained spermatozoa. The 8 agglutinating sera that stained the ejaculated spermatozoa in dilutions of 1:10 or higher also stained testicular spermatozoa. Thus sperm agglutinins are in general antibodies that react with antigens found in testicular spermatozoa. So far no antibodies have been found that react primarily with coating antigens originating from the adnexal glands, so that sperm resorption is likely to be a factor in autoantibody formation.

A long-term investigation has been planned to study the different ways in which sperm might be resorbed in cases showing serum sperm-aggluti-nins. In one of the old people's homes of Amster-dam we have found that, out of 105 male residents born in the past century, 9 had sperm agglutinins in their serum with a titre of 1:32 or higher. As autopsies are done on all deaths, histological surveys of the whole genital tract of these people are planned.

When in a control series of sera of old women we found, to our surprise, that 5 out of 123 women born before 1900 had sperm agglutinins in a titre of 1:32 or higher we wondered about other explanations. A woman suffering from liver cirrhosis, aged 84, had a titre of 1:512. Of course, these women may have true isoantibodies to sperm induced by resorption possibly a long time ago; but it seems more likely that the sperm agglutinins in these cases are cross-reacting anti-bodies induced by other autoantigens or by external antigens such as bacterial substances. We hope that we can solve some of these questions in the near future.

Therapy

Those patients who show complete autoaggluti-nation in their ejaculate have been infertile for as long as we have followed their cases, which for some patients is more than ten years, and so far therapeutic trials have been unsuccessful. ACTH or corticosteroids in moderate doses for a period of two months has not altered their serum titres or the autoagglutination.

Recently we started to treat some men with testosterone, in the hope that antibody formation would diminish after termination of sperm resorption by testosterone-induced suppression of spermatogenesis. If this proves discouraging we plan hemicastration in cases of proved one-sided obstruction to remove the source of excessive resorption.

Some years ago we attempted to elute the auto-antibodies from the agglutinated sperm for the purpose of making it suitable for artificial insemination and found that the semen seemed to be normal after incubation with 1% trypsin for half an hour; the clumps disintegrated while the sperm did not lose motility. But unfortunately pigs inseminated with boar sperm incubated with trypsin showed that this procedure might be harmful to offspring (Rümke 1964).

Acknowledgments: I am grateful to Dr M W Kalff (Leiden) for the quantitative determinations of the immunoglobulins and to Dr F Dekking (Amsterdam) for the antimeasles virus CF tests.

REFERENCES

Burgos M H (1967) *VII Int. Conf. int. planned Parenthood Fed.*, p 342
Feltkamp F E W, Kruyff K, Ladiges N C J J & Rümke P (1965) *Ann. N. Y. Acad. Sci.* 124, 702
Fjällbrant B (1965) *Acta obstet. gynec. scand.* 44, 474
Kibrick S, Belding D L & Merrill B (1952) *Fertil. and Steril.* 3, 430
Mancini R E, Andrada J A, Saraceni D, Bachmann A E, Lavieri J C & Nemirovsky M (1965) *J. clin. Endocr.* 25, 859
Masson P & Heremans J F (1966) In: Molecular Biology of Human Proteins. Ed. H E Schultze & J F Heremans. Amsterdam; 1, 850
Phadke A M (1964) *J. Reprod. Fertil.* 7, 1
Phadke A M & Padukone K (1964) *J. Reprod. Fertil.* 7, 163
Rümke P (1954) *Vox Sang. (Basel)* 4, 135
(1964) *II Int. Congr. Endocr.* p 906
(1965) *Ann. N. Y. Acad. Sci.* 124, 696
Rümke P & Hellinga G (1959) *Amer. J. clin. Path.* 32, 357
Weil A J (1965) *Ann. N. Y. Acad. Sci.* 124, 267
Wilson L (1954) *Proc. Soc. exp. Biol., N. Y.* 85, 652

Voluntary Sterilization in the Male

H. J. Roberts

Your approval of vasectomy as a definitive method of voluntary sterilization (1 June, p. 508) warrants comment and caution. There can be no doubt as to its simplicity and effectiveness. The long-term medical complications of this procedure, however, have yet to be critically evaluated.

This disturbing note of reserve stems from my observations[1] on men in their 20s and 30s who presented with a host of puzzling systemic disorders within one or more years after elective vasectomy. Previously, all had enjoyed apparent good health. The features for which they sought consultation included unexplained thrombophlebitis, prolonged fever, generalized lymph node enlargement, arthropathy, recurrent infection, various skin eruptions, glomerulonephritis, interstitial pulmonary fibrosis, severe narcolepsy, acute multiple sclerosis, liver dysfunction (increased bromsulphalein retention), increased circulating gammaglobulin, and, a biologic false-positive serologic reaction. Aside from reactive hypoglycaemia, the only common denominator was vasectomy. The possible pathogenetic mechanisms have been discussed in the cited paper; they include induced hormonal imbalances, autosensitization to testicular nucleoprotein, and altered blood coagulation. Since my initial report, these findings have been encountered in additional patients. By questioning *every* individual with such unexplained features, a history of vasectomy prior to their onset has been uncovered when it was completely forgotten during routine query about previous surgery.

In view of the vast socio-economic implications of population explosion, it is understandable that these admittedly limited clinical experiences are disturbing to all who recognize the urgent need for its enlightened control, including myself. Failure to pursue the matter by careful analysis of large numbers of vasectomized men, however, may be an invitation to wholesale iatrogenic damage. This is especially pertinent when governments formally encourage and even subsidize such surgery. Restraint also should be exercised when projecting the purported innocuousness of mass vasectomy programmes being conducted in famine-threatened countries on to the populations of relatively affluent countries, because its imunologic and other sequelae may be conditioned by nutrition, other ecologic factors, and hyperinsulinized-diabetic state. In a recent review of vasectomy in India[2] it was pointed out that as many as 80% of the Indian population suffer from "malnutritional dwarfism."

REFERENCES

[1] Roberts, H. J., *J. Amer. Geriat. Soc.*, 1968, **16**, 267.
[2] Keatley, R., *Wall Street Journal*, 1968, **172**, No. 10, p. 1.

SPERMAGGLUTININ FORMATION IN MALE RATS BY SUBCUTANEOUSLY INJECTED SYNGENEIC EPIDIDYMAL SPERMATOZOA AND BY VASOLIGATION OR VASECTOMY

PH. RÜMKE AND M. TITUS

INTRODUCTION

Infertility due to auto-immunity to spermatozoa occurs in animals under experimental, and in the human male under natural, conditions. In experimental systems, immunization with spermatozoa or testis extracts, incorporated in complete Freund's adjuvant, leads to an auto-allergic orchitis which manifests itself clinically in the disappearance of spermatozoa from the ejaculate and aspermatogenesis (reviewed by Voisin & Toullet, 1968). When the same antigens are injected with incomplete Freund's adjuvant (i.e. without the killed mycobacteria), the animals will only develop antibodies against spermatozoa, but their testes will not be affected. It is surprising that there are no reports concerning the reproductive function of animals with antibodies against spermatozoa but with normal testis histology; the more so since it is known that, in the case of the infertile male patient, auto-antibodies against spermatozoa can render them incapable of fertilization, and this often occurs in patients with normal testicular histology and a normal production of spermatozoa (Rümke & Hellinga, 1959; Fjällbrant, 1965, 1968). The disparity between what is known about the experimental animal and about the human patient is emphasized by the fact that spermagglutinins are the antibodies least looked for in animals immunized with spermatozoa or testis extracts whereas in men spermagglutinins, and also immobilizing antibodies, play an important rôle in infertility.

The history and physical examination of such patients often suggest that some of their spermatozoa were or are continuously resorbed either in the epididymis or rete testis, as, for example, when a patient has an obstruction in his efferent ducts (Rümke, 1965). Various reports on series of patients with obstructions reveal that about a quarter of such individuals have spermagglutinins in their serum (Phadke, 1964; Rümke, 1967). Information about sperm auto-antibody (especially spermagglutinin) formation after vasoligation in animals is limited. Only Bratanov, Dikov & Popova (1964) claimed that, after unilateral ligation of the vas deferens in the rabbit, ram and bull, spermagglutinins may develop.

The present study aimed to show that: (1) the macroscopic agglutination technique as described by Kibrick, Belding & Merrill (1952), and used by us for the titration of spermagglutinins in human sera, could well be used in a modified form for the detection and titration of spermagglutinins in rat serum against rat spermatozoa; (2) male rats injected with large amounts of epididymal spermatozoa of the same strain develop spermagglutinins; (3) vasoligation or vasectomy in the rat can lead to the formation of auto-spermagglutinins as in man; and (4) serum-spermagglutinins, as such, do not interfere with spermatogenesis and do not necessarily impair the fertility of the animals.

MATERIALS AND METHODS

Rats

Male rats of the inbred (sixty generations) Wistar line, called R-strain, of the stock of the Netherlands Cancer Institute were used for all experiments. All procedures were performed in a room with a constant temperature of 30° C.

Sperm suspensions

Epididymal spermatozoa were collected from rats exsanguinated under ether anaesthesia by dissecting the epididymis and vas deferens free of blood vessels, and mincing them with scissors in medium in a watch glass. Motile spermatozoa swam out of the minced pieces into the medium, giving it a milky appearance within a few minutes. This sperm suspension was transferred through a wide-mouth pipette (care being taken to avoid air bubbles) into a measuring glass where it was pooled with the suspensions derived from other rats. The medium was added to the pool so that the final sperm concentration was of the order of 10^7 spermatozoa/ml, and such a suspension could be used for the sperm-agglutination test. The medium, a modified Hanks's solution, consisted of 8 g NaCl, 0·4 g KCl, 1 g glucose, 0·5 ml $MgSO_4.7H_2O$ 40%, 0·5 ml KH_2PO_4

12%, 0·5 ml Na$_2$HPO$_4$.2H$_2$O 12%, 4 ml NaHCO$_3$ 5%, and 5 g bovine lact-albuminhydrolysate, with water added to make 1 litre; the pH was 6·7 to 6·9.

When spermatozoa were to be used for immunization procedures, they were suspended in phosphate-buffered saline solution (pH 7·4) instead of the modified Hanks's solution.

Spermagglutination test

The spermagglutination test was performed (without using gelatin) according to a modification of the technique of Kibrick, Belding & Merrill (1952). The rat sera to be tested were heated for 30 min at 56° C, since unheated serum immobilizes spermatozoa nonspecifically. Dilutions were made with the same medium that was used to suspend the spermatozoa. Volumes of 0·3 ml were placed in small glass tubes with internal diameters of 6 mm. The same volume of the stock sperm suspension (10^7 spermatozoa/ml) was added, and serum and spermatozoa were mixed as gently as possible. The tubes were left in the same room at 30° C, and readings were taken macroscopically after 1, 2 and 3 hr. The granular appearance of the agglutination reaction can be clearly distinguished from the homogeneous appearance of the negative reaction.

Immunization procedures

Rats to be immunized with syngeneic spermatozoa were injected subcutaneously with different amounts of unwashed epididymal spermatozoa suspended in phosphate-buffered saline. In a few experiments, complete and incomplete Freund's adjuvant (Difco) were used. The immunization schedules are given under the heading of the experiments.

Vasoligation and vasectomy

These surgical procedures were always performed on only one side (the left). The instruments were clean, but not sterile. After incising the cutaneous and muscular layers on the ventral surface along the penis, the vas deferens was dissected free of blood vessels for approximately 1 cm. For a vasectomy, that part which had been dissected free was cut out and removed, the remaining ends not being closed. For a vasoligation, the same operation was performed, except that ligatures were first placed on the vas at either side of the two places where the vas was to be transected.

Serum

After general anaesthesia with ether, rats were bled to death from the carotid artery. When the animal was kept alive, 1 to 2 ml blood was drawn from an orbital vein. After clotting and centrifugation, serum was separated and stored at −20° C.

Fertility test

The male to be tested was placed with a virgin female rat which, according to the vaginal smear pattern, exhibited regular oestrous cycles. If, after 32 days, the female was not yet pregnant, she was replaced by another female

of proven fertility. The male rat was considered to be sterile when the secon
female also did not become pregnant after 32 days.

EXPERIMENTS AND RESULTS

Experiments to standardize the spermagglutination test
The macroscopic spermagglutination test, as described by Kibrick *et al.*
(1952), is routinely used in this laboratory for the detection of spermagglutinins
in human sera. The same technique using rat epididymal spermatozoa was

TABLE 1

EFFECTS OF SPERM CONCENTRATION AND TEMPERATURE ON SPERM-
AGGLUTINATION

Incubation temp.	Sperm conc. $\times 10^6/ml$	Normal serum dilutions			Immune serum dilutions		
		1:90	1:270	1:810	1:90	1:270	1:810
20° C	20	±	±	±	±	±	±
	10	—	—	—	—	—	—
	5	—	—	—	—	—	—
	2·5	—	—	—	—	—	—
27° C	20	±	±	±	±	±	±
	10	—	—	—	+	+	—
	5	—	—	—	+	+	—
	2·5	—	—	—	+	—	—
30° C	20	±	±	±	±	±	±
	10	—	—	—	+	+	+
	5	—	—	—	+	+	—
	2·5	—	—	—	+	+	—
37° C	20	±	±	±	±	±	±
	10	—	—	—	+	—	—
	5	—	—	—	+	—	—
	2·5	—	—	—	—	—	—

tried for the testing of rat sera, but, in contrast to human spermatozoa, rat
spermatozoa were found to lose their motility in phosphate-buffered glucose
gelatin solution, and were not therefore suitable for the spermagglutination test
since this always needs spermatozoa of good motility. However, when this
medium was replaced by a modified Hanks's solution (see 'Materials') without
gelatin, the rat spermatozoa retained their motility for several hours, and were
easily agglutinated by a rat antiserum against spermatozoa, whereas the normal
sera of untreated young adult rats did not agglutinate the spermatozoa, provided they were inactivated by heating to 56° C for 30 min. Unheated sera
showed immobilization and/or pseudoagglutination.

.For further standardization experiments, a normal serum and a serum
sample from a rat immunized with epididymal rat spermatozoa were used.
Agglutination tests were performed at different incubation temperatures and
with sperm suspensions of different concentrations (see Table 1).

With a stock sperm suspension of 2×10^7 spermatozoa/ml, the readings were
difficult since with all serum dilutions and temperatures the macroscopic
appearance of the control showed a rather broken, as contrasted with a homo-

geneous, turbidity. With sperm concentrations of 1×10^7/ml or less, the controls were homogeneous, indicating total absence of macroscopic agglutination. The immune serum readings were best with a concentration of 1×10^7/ml. The titre was higher with that concentration than with 0·5 and 0·25 $\times 10^7$/ml.

The incubation temperature of 30° C gave the best results. This was also to be expected from the fact that, at 30° C, the motility of the spermatozoa lasted the longest. Therefore, all further tests were performed at 30° C with a suspension concentration of 10^7 spermatozoa/ml.

Readings were made after 1, 2 and 3 hr since weak spermagglutinating sera could show agglutination only after 3 hr, but stronger sera acted in such a short time that, after 1 hr, the clumps of spermatozoa settled down in the bottom of the tube, making the reading less clear. Therefore, it seemed advisable to take readings also after 1 and 2 hr.

Sera of young adult male rats generally did not show agglutination within 3 hr.

That the test was capable of yielding highly reproducible results was shown by seven spermagglutinating sera which were re-tested after an interval of about 5 months, during which the sera were kept at $-20°$ C. The titres of the first and second tests with each serum were 1280–1280, 1280–640, 640–640, 640–640, 320–320, 320–320 and 40–40, respectively. The titres at the second test were read by one of us (M.T.) without knowledge of the results of the first test.

Naturally occurring spermagglutinins in male rats

For the immunization experiments described below, the sera of thirty-six animals were tested when they were $3\frac{1}{2}$ months old, several months before the experiment started. One of these animals possessed spermagglutinins in the serum in a titre of 20; the others were all negative at a dilution of 1:5. Two out of eight untreated control animals for another experiment (auto-immunization by vasoligation or vasectomy) had low titres (5 and 10) when they were nearly 1 year old. In the beginning of this experiment, none of the twenty-three male rats possessed spermagglutinins in their serum. In another series, sera were tested from fifteen male rats 283 to 330 days old. The sera of six rats in a dilution of 1:5 were negative, three were positive with a titre of 5, and six with a titre of 10.

It can thus be stated that titres of 40 or higher never occurred under natural conditions in seventy-four male rats of various ages.

Immunization experiments

Seven-month-old male rats were given four subcutaneous injections with syngeneic epididymal spermatozoa according to the scheme given in Text-fig. 1. Spermagglutinin titres were detected in blood drawn 7, 14, 21, 28 and 47 days after the first injection. As shown in Text-fig. 1, the six rats injected with the highest amount, i.e. 1·5 to 2·3 $\times 10^9$ spermatozoa/rat, responded within 7 days after one injection with titres of 640 to 2560. The second group, which received ten times less than the first, responded less vigorously. Only one animal attained a titre of 640, but this animal had a titre of 20 before the

124

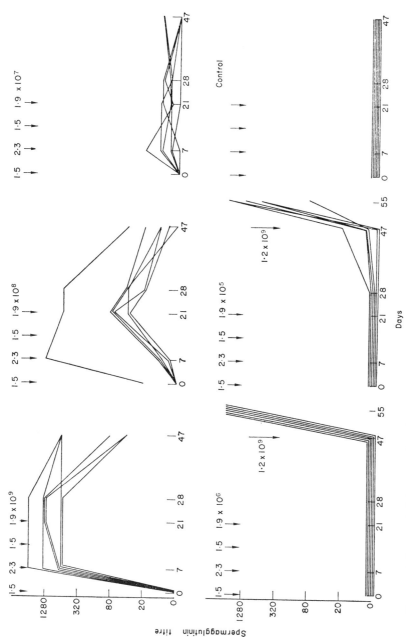

TEXT-FIG. 1. Spermagglutinin response in male rats to subcutaneously injected syngeneic epididymal rat spermatozoa (six rats per group).

125

experiment started; the others did not reach higher than 80 on the 21st day after having received three injections. All titres declined in the 4 weeks after the last injection. The rats which received 10^7 spermatozoa/injection never developed titres higher than 20. The rats of the other groups did not respond at all.

Since the question arose as to whether injection of low doses rendered the animals tolerant, the rats which had received 10^6 and 10^5 spermatozoa/injection were injected with 10^9 spermatozoa after 47 days. All rats had sperm-agglutinin titres 7 days later which were as high as those of the first group which received 10^9 spermatozoa on the first day of the experiment. From this, it follows that doses of 10^6 and 10^5 spermatozoa were too low to stimulate spermagglutinin formation, and that the animals were not rendered tolerant by these low doses.

Auto-immunization by unilateral vasoligation or vasectomy

Unilateral vasoligation was performed on seven rats and unilateral vasec-tomy on eight rats. Eight control rats underwent a sham operation. All rats were of the same age and strain. Blood was taken just before, and 113, 165 and 215 days after, operation. As shown in Text-fig. 2, two of the eight control rats had, on the 215th day, spermagglutinins in titres of 5 and 10, similar to titres acquired spontaneously with age. However, out of the seven vasoligated animals, two developed high spermagglutinin titres (1280 and 640 on the 215th day), while five had low titres (not higher than 10). All eight vasectom-ized rats developed titres ranging from 40 to 1280 (five of them had a titre of 320 or higher).

Thus two of seven vasoligated rats and all eight vasectomized rats developed spermagglutinins in titres higher than were ever encountered under natural conditions. It is striking that more vasectomized than vasoligated animals reacted, presumably because the spermatozoa of the vasectomized rats were free to flow into the peritoneal cavity.

All rats involved in this experiment were proved to be fertile within the first 10 days after the operation, showing that the non-operated side was function-ally normal. On the 197th day, they were tested again for their capacity to fertilize. Of the two vasoligated rats with high titres, the one with a sperm-agglutinin titre of 1280 on the 215th day appeared to be fertile, while the other, with a titre of 640, was sterile. The vasoligated rats with low titres were all fertile, as was the vasectomized rat with a titre of 1280; four other fertile rats had titres of 320, 160, 80 and 40. Three rats, all with titres of 640 on the 215th day, were sterile. These observations show that the autospermagglutinins as such are not necessarily impairing the fertility of the male rat. If continuous resorption of spermatozoa on the operated side was responsible for a lasting spermagglutinin titre, a hemicastration on the operated side would lead to a decrease of the titre. Four animals of the group of the vasectomized rats were, therefore, hemicastrated and four others of the same group had a sham operation (laparotomy). For the hemicastration, animals with titres of 1280, 640, 640 and 160, and for the sham operation, animals with titres of 640, 320, 80 and 40, on the 215th day, were chosen. Hemicastration was carried out on the same

126

side of the abdomen as the vasectomy, the testis was pulled into the peritoneal cavity, the blood vessels were ligated, and the testis, epididymis and vas deferens peripheral to the vasectomy were extirpated.

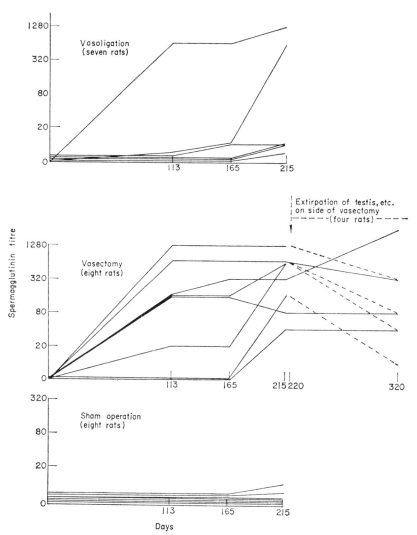

TEXT-FIG. 2. Spermagglutinin formation after vasoligation or vasectomy.

Animals were bled 95 days after the operation. All four hemicastrated animals showed a significant drop in titre (1280 to 320, 640 to 80, 640 to 40, 160 to 10). The sham-operated rats did not show any significant decrease in titre (640 to 320, 320 to 2560, 80 to 80, 40 to 40). The results suggest that

127

removal of the source of antibody stimulation leads to a gradual disappearance of the antibodies.

Since only two out of the seven vasoligated rats developed spermagglutinins in high titres, the other five might have been rendered tolerant. This possibility was tested by injecting all seven animals subcutaneously with $1 \cdot 2 \times 10^6$ spermatozoa on the 215th day. Eight days later, the titres were changed respectively from 1280 to 640, 640 to 40, 10 to 1280, 10 to 320, 10 to 320, 5 to 1280 and 0 to 640. With the exception of the second animal, which showed a sharp decrease in titre (for which we have no explanation), all animals appeared to react to the relatively small dose of 10^6 spermatozoa, and thus were not tolerant. On the contrary, the low titres apparently reflected a state of continuous low stimulation, and the dose of 10^6 spermatozoa, which was insufficient to stimulate spermagglutinin formation in non-treated animals (see Text-fig. 1), acted here, presumably, as a booster injection initiating a secondary response.

Pathology of the vasoligated or vasectomized rats

The vasoligated rats were killed on the 231st day, 16 days after they received the injection of 10^6 spermatozoa. The testis on the non-operated right side was macroscopically normal or even slightly enlarged in all seven animals; the epididymis contained normal motile spermatozoa on that side, and microscopically too, these testes showed no abnormalities.

Two animals that both possessed titres of 10 on the 215th day had normal testes on the operated left side, and the vas and epididymis contained normal motile spermatozoa. The blind end of the vas deferens ended in a 'pocket' built up by the peritoneum. It contained sperm tails, which had apparently leaked through the ligated and necrotic vas. All other rats of this group had signs of degeneration of the left testis, and the vas and epididymis contained headless and immotile spermatozoa.

The testes of the vasectomized animals were either investigated at the time when four of the animals were hemicastrated, or after the experiment when they had a sham operation. In all eight cases, the right testes were normal or slightly enlarged with normal motile spermatozoa in the right vas. The left testes all showed signs of degeneration, always with headless immotile spermatozoa in the vas. Histologically there was considerable degeneration of the testes on the left side.

The testes of the animals immunized with spermatozoa without Freund's adjuvant all appeared to be normal, with normal spermatozoa in the vas when they were killed 78 days after the beginning of the experiment. The four rats immunized with spermatozoa emulsified in Freund's adjuvant had testes with histological signs of degeneration on both sides (72 days after the first and only injection of spermatozoa in complete Freund's adjuvant).

DISCUSSION

The results show that the macroscopic agglutination technique as described by Kibrick *et al.* (1952) is a very suitable technique for the detection of antibodies against spermatozoa, e.g. spermagglutinins in rat serum. Prerequisites are the gentle handling of the epididymal spermatozoa, an appropriate medium and a constant temperature of 30° C. It is a sensitive technique and easily reproducible. The highest titre ever found with a serum of an immunized male rat was 2560.

Occasionally, the sera of untreated male animals (especially when they were old) possessed spermagglutinins, but never in titres higher than 20.

The immunization experiments showed that male rats can be immunized with syngeneic epididymal spermatozoa, even without the use of an adjuvant, provided that a sufficiently high dose is used. Immunization with epididymal spermatozoa seems to be a matter of quantity rather than quality since this finding has demonstrated the auto-antigenicity of epididymal spermatozoa before they mix with the secretions of the adnexal glands.

The experiments with unilaterally vasoligated or vasectomized rats show that spermatozoa, when abnormally resorbed, can induce the formation of spermagglutinins. However, not all vasoligated animals developed sperm-agglutinins (at least, not in high titres). Those animals with the lower titres, or even without detectable spermagglutinins, developed high titres 1 week after they were injected subcutaneously with 10^6 spermatozoa although this dose had been found to be too low to stimulate spermagglutinin formation in normal, untreated animals. Thus, it seems reasonable to assume that this dose is enough to stimulate high agglutinin production in an animal already 'primed' by continuous resorption of low doses of spermatozoa.

That the vasoligated animals responded diversely might be the result of variations in two factors. In the first place, since the operations were not carried out under sterile conditions, it could well be that bacterial infections were potentiating an antibody response to the sperm antigens. On the other hand, infections and vascular lesions could disturb the spermatogenesis of the testis on the affected side when too few spermatozoa might be resorbed to stimulate spermagglutinin formation. The validity of these suppositions was not further investigated in the current experiments.

An important finding was that male rats remained fertile with high titres (1280) of spermagglutinins. The agglutinins apparently did not enter the control testis which remained normal histologically, and they either did not enter the seminal fluid, or entered but failed to impair the fertilizing ability of the spermatozoa. It is not known if the failure of the agglutinins to enter the seminal plasma is a feature of the species or if the antibody globulin was non-penetrating IgM. In man, IgG and IgA are found in seminal plasma, but not IgM.

Mancini, Vilar, Alvarez & Seiguer (1964) claimed that, in the rat, serum proteins may diffuse from the blood into the tubular lumini of the testis. They did not state, however, whether there is a difference in this respect between macroglobulins and other globulins. Possibly spermagglutinins in our fertile animals are IgM antibodies, that would leave the testis unaffected if they were unable to diffuse from the blood.

It is surprising how little is known about the presence of sperm antibodies in semen of animals known to have such antibodies in the blood following auto-

129

immunization procedures. The observation of Wentworth & Mellen (1964) that Japanese quails immunized with testicular spermatozoa had agglutinated spermatozoa in the vas deferens, is unique in this respect.

A few rats with spermagglutinins were sterile in spite of repeated attempts to prove their fertility, and in spite of proven fertility just after vasoligation or vasectomy. Their testes on the non-operated sides were normal. It seems possible that, in these cases, sperm antibodies do reach the seminal fluid. But no further attempt has been made to characterize the spermagglutinins according to their antibody type.

Finally, the finding that the spermagglutinin titre decreased after extirpation of the affected epididymis and testis illustrated that a continuous resorption of sperm antigens seemed necessary for a lasting spermagglutinin titre.

ACKNOWLEDGMENTS

This investigation received financial support from the World Health Organization.

REFERENCES

BRATANOV, K., DIKOV, V. & POPOVA, Y. (1964) Sur la formation des auto-spermo-anticorps chez les reproduceurs. *C.r. Acad. bulg. Sci.* **17,** 1117.

FJÄLLBRANT, B. (1965) Immunoagglutination of sperm in cases of sterility. *Acta obst. gynec. scand.* **44,** 474.

FJÄLLBRANT, B. (1968) Sperm antibodies and sterility in men. *Acta obst. gynec. scand.* **47,** Suppl. **4,** 38.

KIBRICK, S., BELDING, D. L. & MERRILL, B. (1952) Methods for the detection of antibodies against mammalian spermatozoa. *Fert. Steril.* **3,** 419 and 430.

MANCINI, R. E., VILAR, O., ALVAREZ, B. & SEIGUER, A. C. (1964) Extravascular and intratubular diffusion of labeled serum proteins in the rat testis. *J. Histochem. Cytochem.* **13,** 376.

PHADKE, A. M. (1964) Fate of spermatozoa in case of obstructive azoospermia and after ligation of vas deferens in man. *J. Reprod. Fert.* **7,** 1.

RÜMKE, PH. (1965) Autospermagglutinins: A cause of infertility in men. *Ann. N.Y. Acad. Sci.* **124,** 696.

RÜMKE PH. (1967) Sperm-agglutinating autoantibodies in relation to male infertility. *Proc. R. Soc. Med.* **61,** 275.

RÜMKE, PH. & HELLINGA, G. (1959) Auto-antibodies against spermatozoa in sterile men. *Am. J. clin. Path.* **32,** 357.

VOISIN, G. A. & TOULLET, F. (1968) Étude sur l'orchite aspermatogénétique autoimmune et les autoantigènes de spermatozoïdes chez le cobaye. *Annls Inst. Pasteur, Paris,* **114,** 727.

WENTWORTH, B. C. & MELLEN, W. J. (1964) Active immunity induced and spermatogenesis suppressed by testicular antigen in the male Japanese quail. *J. Reprod. Fert.* **8,** 215.

DELAYED THROMBOPHLEBITIS AND SYSTEMIC COMPLICATIONS AFTER VASECTOMY: POSSIBLE ROLE OF DIABETOGENIC HYPERINSULINISM

H. J. ROBERTS, M.D.

There has been accelerated interest by governments, individuals, and the medical profession concerning the socio-economic implications of the current population explosion and its enlightened control. As recognition of the serious side effects and other limitations of "birth-control" pills and intra-uterine devices becomes more widespread, the prevention of conception by surgical and pharmacologic methods directed primarily to males will receive increased attention. Many physicians and patients are currently enthusiastic over the effectiveness, convenience, and presumed harmless nature of elective vasectomy. In 1964, Guttmacher (1) deduced that approximately 45,000 vasectomies were being performed annually in the United States for the purpose of family limitation. Indeed, it has been estimated that 7 per cent of the husbands of fertile wives in the southwestern United States had undergone vasectomy by 1960 (2).

As a medical consultant without previous professional or other bias against vasectomy, I have become increasingly concerned relative to several possible serious systemic complications of the procedure, especially when performed on well-nourished young men who are subject to the chronic hyperinsulinized state (diabetogenic hyperinsulinism). This state is tending to become a hallmark of our culture, largely owing to nutritional developments since the turn of the century (3–5). These misgivings are further heightened by the immunologic consequences of experimental vasectomy and related procedures.

The clinical experiences to be presented might prove coincidental in a consultation practice that is admittedly atypical. They nevertheless pose a sobering perspective that calls for clarification by careful long-term statistical studies conducted on significant numbers of vasectomized men, if enormous iatrogenic damage by ill-advised wholesale vasectomy is to be averted. Failure to have recognized these complications can be understood in the light of their delayed nature, their extragenital manifestations, and the absence of comparable previous reports in the literature.

THROMBOPHLEBITIS

Three men in the fourth age decade have been observed in whom thrombophlebitis developed months or years following vasectomy. The attacks could not be explained on conventional grounds, i.e., precipitation by local trauma, or excessive standing or squatting. Owing to the prolonged intervals after surgery, such phlebitis could not be reasonably regarded as local complications of the operative procedure.

Case 1. This 33-year-old white engineer was hospitalized for acute thrombophlebitis in the left lower extremity, of several weeks' duration. No unusual activities that might have precipitated the attack could be recalled. A bilateral vasectomy had been performed eighteen months previously. His history was also characterized by severe hypoglycemic features with a recurrent craving for sweets, pathologic drowsiness, and migrainous headaches.

On physical examination the findings were normal except for tenderness and induration over the deep calf vein. The patient was not obese. No underlying systemic disorder could be uncovered by extensive study. A randomly determined blood glucose concentration (Folin-Wu) at 4:15 p.m. was 63 mg per 100 ml. The results (Auto-Analyzer) of glucose tolerance testing were as follows: fasting, 86 mg; half hour, 120 mg; one hour, 109 mg; two hours, 93 mg; three hours, 74 mg; and four hours, 71 mg per 100 ml.

The patient was treated with local soaks, heparin and oral anticoagulants. The thrombophlebitis improved slowly over a three-month period.

Case 2. This 36-year-old executive had enjoyed apparent excellent health. A vasectomy was performed in June 1967, largely owing to the fact that his wife was debilitated with chronic hepatitis. After doing well for two months, he experienced unexplained severe anterior chest pain. He was seen by another physician, who administered an opiate and entertained the diagnosis of acute coronary insufficiency. When seen two weeks later, there were nonspecific changes both in the chest x-ray films and the electrocardiogram. Further questioning indicated a definite pleuritic component in the chest pain. He subsequently experienced a comparable attack in two weeks, which was diagnosed as probable pulmonary embolism. Tenderness was elicited over the deep vein of the left calf. The patient was then queried specifically concerning previous vasectomy, at which point the foregoing surgical history was obtained. In view of his recurrent embolic attacks, oral anticoagulant therapy was started. There has been no recurrence of the attacks over the ensuing four months.

Another 36-year-old male, vasectomized four years previously, noted the onset of an unexplained and progressively larger varicosity in the right lower extremity about two years postoperatively. There was no frank clinical attack of thrombophlebitis.

OTHER SYSTEMIC COMPLICATIONS

Three vasectomized men have been observed who presented serious and puzzling systemic features. Their disorders were characterized by varying combinations of prolonged fever, generalized lymph node enlargement, various eruptions, arthropathy, recurrent infections, glomerulonephritis, interstitial pulmonary fibrosis, neuropsychiatric aberrations, an elevated level of circulating globulins, elevated BSP retention, and a biologic false-positive serologic reaction. Although such disorders as systemic lupus erythematosus, occult lymphoma, sarcoidosis, primary tuberculosis, Whipple's disease, chronic hepatitis, and other connective tissue or vascular diseases were seriously considered in the differential diagnosis, their presence could not be definitively established. In another patient, acute multiple sclerosis developed several months after a vasectomy.

Case 3. A 36-year-old white postman was seen in consultation because of a 20-pound weight loss in recent months, recurrent infections, peptic-ulcer-like symptoms, recurrent lymph node enlargement (previously thought to be "recurrent infectious mononucleosis" or cat-scratch infection), severe weakness, and profuse sweats. He had undergone vasectomy two years previously. There was a past history of duodenitis. The pertinent findings on physical examination included evidence of weight loss, bilaterally enlarged cervical lymph nodes, acute prostatitis, and a somewhat enlarged and tender left testicle.

The leukocyte count was 16,600 per cu mm, with 44% segmented polymorphonuclear cells, 52% lymphocytes, and 4% eosinophils. The results (AutoAnalyzer) of glucose tolerance testing were as follows: fasting, 72 mg; half hour, 175 mg; one hour, 208 mg; two hours, 183 mg; three hours, 60 mg; and four hours, 66 mg per 100 ml. Results of numerous other studies were normal. These tests included the remaining blood indices, urinalysis, serum calcium and phosphorus concentrations, transaminase activity, BSP retention, blood protein electrophoresis, serologic reactions for lues, LE cell preparations, a rheumatoid arthritis (RA) test, quantitative urinary excretion of adrenocortical steroids, intermediate-strength PPD (for tuberculosis) and histoplasmin skin tests, an electrocardiogram, and multiple roentgenograms. Serologic tests for the lymphogranuloma venereum group of virus infections also gave negative results.

133

The patient was treated symptomatically with diet and decreasing amounts of dexamethasone orally. He gained 11 pounds. A subsequent flareup of the prostatitis and seminal vesiculitis responded to an increased dosage of steroid therapy, and tetracycline. This patient could be observed for only two months.

Case 4. A 32-year-old white automobile mechanic was seen in consultation for a complex clinical problem involving considerable recent weight loss, recurrent fever (as high as 102° F during the afternoon) over a period of several months, erythema multiforme, recurrent petechiae and hives, repeated infections of the sinuses and bronchial tubes, acute prostatitis necessitating urologic treatment, intermittent diarrhea, aching of the joints, severe headaches with migrainous scotomata, generalized lymph node enlargement, and increasing nervousness. A vasectomy had been performed several years previously. There was a past history of acute pancreatitis. A maternal relative was diabetic.

The pertinent findings on physical examination included generalized lymph node enlargement, a low-grade fever, bilateral asthmatic breath sounds, enlargement and tenderness of the prostate, two café-au-lait spots, and multiple petechiae. An active duodenal ulcer was found subsequently.

He was studied extensively not only during three hospital admissions locally, but also at two university centers. The possibility of Whipple's disease was seriously entertained, but could not be verified by lymph node or intestinal biopsy (John Hopkins Hospital). The pertinent laboratory findings included a biologic false-positive serologic reaction, negative results with the intermediate-strength PPD skin test for tuberculosis, the presence of nonspecific reactive hyperplasia in multiple lymph node biopsy specimens obtained during two admissions, and blood glucose levels indicating reactive hypoglycemia. The results (AutoAnalyzer) of glucose tolerance testing were as follows: fasting, 82 mg; half hour, 149 mg; one hour, 177 mg; two hours, 115 mg; three hours, 52 mg; and four hours, 80 mg per 100 ml. Numerous blood cultures at each institution, including a search for anaerobic and atypical bacteria, failed to uncover any organisms. A small bronchiectatic area was noted by bronchography. X-ray studies of the gastrointestinal tract and kidneys were not remarkable. Examination showed the bone marrow to be essentially normal. BSP retention (45 minutes) was 1.2 per cent. One serum lactic dehydrogenase determination was high (710 units). Protein electrophoretic studies, multiple LE cell preparations and an RA test were within normal limits. Liver biopsy failed to disclose any granulomatous or other contributory pathologic process. Studies of adrenocortical function yielded normal results.

Over an 18-month period of careful observation, the patient was treated symptomatically as far as possible for recurrent infections involving many organs, the cited active duodenal ulcer, marked nervousness, and a severe attack of labyrinthitis. (There was insufficient evidence to warrant a diagnosis of brain abscess.) Numerous antibiotics and other supportive measures, including frequent injections of gamma globulin, administration of adrenocortical steroids orally and parenterally, multivitamins, several courses of aerosol therapy, cessation of smoking, and a trial of antituberculosis management failed to produce a remission.

Case 5. A 48-year-old white financier was seen in consultation for increasingly severe complaints. They included profound fatigue and drowsiness, headache, recurrent sweats, insomnia and abdominal bloat. A vasectomy had been performed one year previously. He smoked approximately ten cigarettes daily.

The initial physical examination was not remarkable. He had never been obese. His blood pressure was 130/90 mm Hg. The electrocardiogram was normal. The hemoglobin level was 12.5 gm per cent, hematocrit 40 per cent, and erythrocyte count 4,190,000 per cu mm. The initial urinalysis also gave normal results. The concentration of blood urea nitrogen was 15 mg per 100 ml, butanol-extractable iodine 4.8 μg per

100 ml, and serum cholesterol 165 mg per 100 ml. In two blood samples obtained randomly in the afternoon, the glucose concentrations were 47 and 53 mg per 100 ml (Folin-Wu). Although the results of morning glucose tolerance testing were not of the diabetic type, there was a hypoglycemic drop at four and a half hours, with associated symptoms. BSP retention (45 minutes) was 7.5 per cent. Chest x-ray films revealed a cardiothoracic ratio of 14.5/30.2 and increased bronchovascular markings.

The patient was treated symptomatically with an antihypoglycemic diet, methylphenidate (Ritalin) and vitamins. In spite of dietary salt restriction, his blood pressure rose progressively over the ensuing months to 136/104, 150/102, 170/130, and 170/130. There was little improvement of the hypertension or headaches during treatment with benzthiazide (Exna) and other antihypertensive measures. In the ensuing year, he experienced repeated gastrointestinal, respiratory and sinus infections, the latter necessitating treatment by an otolaryngologist. The next manifestations were gross hematuria, anemia, an increase in BSP retention (13.7 per cent at 45 minutes), and an increase in the size of the left ventricle. A progressively severe cough and dyspnea on exertion were accompanied by bilateral congestive and fibrotic changes in the lungs. The blood pressure rose to 200/124, but the blood urea nitrogen level remained normal. Intravenous urograms were within normal limits. Antibiotics, adrenocortical steroids and antihypertensive drugs were given, but without appreciable benefit. The patient left the community in March 1966, and has not been seen since. A friend stated that he had been hospitalized one year later for a presumed heart attack.

Case 6. This 45-year-old executive was seen in consultation during November 1967 for progressive multiple sclerosis. The diagnosis first was made in 1961, approximately six months after an uncomplicated elective vasectomy. The typical neurologic features of this disorder were found, including Babinski responses and ankle clonus. Since 1964, there had also been pathologic drowsiness, cataplexy, severe leg cramps, "restless legs" and impotence. He ingested "cokes" frequently to satisfy his recurrent intense desire for sweets. The results (true glucose) of glucose tolerance testing were as follows: fasting, 88 mg; half hour, 146 mg; 1 hour, 127 mg; 2 hours, 97 mg; 3 hours, 65 mg; and 4 hours, 59 mg per 100 ml. Other evidences of the hyperinsulinized diabetic state included a mature left cataract and a blood uric acid concentration of 6.85 mg per 100 ml.

DISCUSSION

When confronted by a relatively young couple who have several children and are seeking counsel about contraception, the conscientious and conservative physician—aware of the many shortcomings and potential hazards of presently available birth-control pills and devices—understandingly may be enthusiastic in recommending vasectomy (6). Unfortunately, our experience would suggest that such a recommendation might carry long-term risks, especially in men who are prone to thrombophlebitis and diabetogenic hyperinsulinism. A recent editorial in the British Medical Journal (7) aptly cautioned: "It is a sound guiding principle of surgery never to disturb the function of a normal structure except as may be necessary for the effective treatment of a related disorder. . . . Consequently, whereas vasectomy may be appropriate in the treatment of established urogenital disease to prevent the spread of infection, its performance in a healthy man for a purpose other than for the protection of his own health is difficult to reconcile with the traditions that normally guide clinical judgement." In a similar vein, Johnson (8) commented: "In short, a major problem with vasectomy is the ease with which it can be and has been used to treat the wrong member of the family. Among our cases the overworked, overfertile housewife seems to be a more suitable candidate for sterilization than does her husband. Nowhere else in medicine do we recommend one procedure when another one is indicated. The ease of performing an inappropriate procedure should not justify doing it."

If delayed *thrombophlebitis* and the cited systemic complications do indeed represent bona fide sequelae of vasectomy, several pathogenetic mechanisms might be involved. They include: 1) inflammatory responses in the male genital tract; 2) gonadotropic and other hormonal imbalances involving the pituitary-testicular "axis," perhaps favoring thrombophlebitis in a manner akin to its recognized precipitation by estrogen-progesterone combinations for birth control; and 3) excessive absorption of testicular proteins and nucleoproteins, with the initiation of an "auto-immune" response. (The concentrated amount of such genetically-involved material is indicated by the fact that the male ejaculate, already largely diluted by secretions from the prostate and seminal vesicles, contains some 400,000,000 spermatozoa in a volume smaller than 0.1 ml) (1). The ability of entrapped sperm to induce considerable inflammation is known to urologists in the form of the occasional severe reaction associated with local seepage after ligation of the duct; at times it resembles a sterile abscess. Moreover, an inflammatory process can be rendered chronic by the development of an auto-immune reaction to one or more of the products of inflammatory exudates (9).

There is also much evidence that *the hyperinsulinized state and diabetes mellitus can alter blood coagulation.* The evidence includes the following:

1. Bridges and associates (10) demonstrated that (a) platelet stickiness was increased in diabetic patients, and (b) the rapid rise in blood glucose concentration (both in normal and diabetic subjects) produced by glucose administration was associated with increased platelet stickiness.

2. Sandberg and associates (11), studying multiple fibrinolytic parameters in diabetic and nondiabetic subjects, found that antifibrinolysin times were much shorter in the diabetic subjects, especially in those receiving 60 or more units of insulin daily. They concluded that such alterations in antifibrinolysin activity reflected the effects of insulin rather than of the diabetic state per se.

3. Mennon (12) suggested that the enhanced fibrinolysis of glucose may constitute an important basis for the empiric use of glucose intravenously in managing acute myocardial infarction. It is of related interest that phenformin and metformin have stimulated fibrinolytic responses in patients with ischemic heart disease and occlusive peripheral vascular disease (13).

4. Skovborg and associates (14, 15) demonstrated a significant increase of blood viscosity in diabetics when compared with controls.

5. Hennes and Awai (16) demonstrated impairment of whole blood and platelets with reference to the formation of fatty acids (especially pal-

mitic acid) in both insulin-independent and insulin-dependent diabetics, primarily affecting renewed synthesis. A possible explanation for such an abnormality is excessive utilization of reduced triphosphopyridine nucleotide by diabetic cells for the reduction of intracellular acetoacetate.

6. The tendency to sludging and sequestration of blood platelets is enhanced by the characteristic microangiopathy in diabetes, particularly the thickening of the capillary basement membrane and endothelial cell proliferation. Whereas basement membrane width in nondiabetic subjects averages 1200 Å (seldom exceeding 1500 Å), the width in diabetics and in diabetic-prone subjects frequently is in the range of 3000 and 8000 Å. Since such basement membrane hypertrophy generally antecedes decreased glucose tolerance in the "prediabetic" group, the writer believes it to be more directly related to the chronic hyperinsulinized state that precedes overt diabetes mellitus.

The *mechanisms of immunopathogenesis in the so-called auto-immune diseases* variously include adsorption of antibody to the surfaces of tissue cells with subsequent sensitization, adsorption of antigen to tissues, phagocytosis of preformed immune complexes, development of specific auto-aggressive antibodies against antigens contained in cell walls, and cellular (rather than humoral) hypersensitivity (17). In disorders such as systemic lupus erythematosus, rheumatoid arthritis and thyroiditis, it is likely that several of these immunologic mechanisms are operative (17). There is increasing evidence to indicate an immunologic potential for DNA (18), even resulting in "DNA autosensitivity." (It is recalled that nucleoprotein consists of nucleic acid linked to a specific protein. RNA is found largely within the cytoplasm of cells, whereas DNA is present almost exclusively in the nucleus.) The rapid response to DNA intradermal skin tests in the reported cases of DNA autosensitivity is impressive (19, 20). The clinical similarities of DNA autosensitivity and systemic lupus erythematosus include ecchymoses, sensitivity to sunlight, renal involvement, hypertension, many nonspecific symptoms (fever, malaise, fatigue, muscle pain, headaches, arthralgia), and a favorable response to antimalarial drugs (19, 20).

Concerning *sensitization to testicular tissue*, the following observations are germane:

1. Since the turn of the century, it has been known that sperm-immobilizing antibodies can be experimentally induced by the intraperitoneal injection of heterologous sperm (21).

2. Wilson (22) and Rümke (23) reported that (a) massive autoagglutination of spermatozoa from infertile men occurred in their seminal plasma, and (b) their blood serum agglutinated donor semen.

3. Freund and associates (24–26), using testicular tissue or spermatozoa combined with adjuvant, demonstrated that sensitization may occur in the guinea pig and rat. There ensued a sloughing of germinal cells, azoospermia, and the development of complement-fixing antibodies and skin sensitization.

137

4. Mancini and associates (27), investigating the immunologic and testicular responses in man, found that auto- or homologous sensitization could be induced in humans with the use of human testicular homogenate plus complete Freund's adjuvant. These responses, presumably representing an induced allergic reaction, were evidenced by the parallel immunologic, histologic, and histo-immunologic findings. Freund and associates also were impressed by the rapidity with which extratubular gonadal changes occurred following cutaneous injection of testicular tissue and adjuvants; engorgement of the blood vessels and edema of the intertubular connective tissue were observed as early as the first day after injection. Perivascular cuffing "resembling periarteritis nodosa" ensued, with infiltration of the intertubular spaces by large mononuclear cells and lymphocytes.

5. Riera and associates (28) demonstrated that the immunization of rabbits with either rabbit semen ejaculate or seminal plasma (incorporated into complete Freund's adjuvant) stimulated the production of antibodies, detectable both by tanned cell hemagglutination and by gel diffusion. Furthermore, the antibody to seminal plasma was shown to be an auto-antibody, which reacted only with seminal plasma and extracts of the accessory glands of reproduction.

6. Yachnin (29) found that heat-denatured bovine serum albumin, in the presence of polynucleotides, is endowed with antigenic properties not exhibited by heat-denatured bovine serum albumin in the absence of polynucleotides. This observation is relevant because of the content of seminal fluid.

In view of the reported recanalization and reversibility following attempted vasectomy (7), the further issue is raised as to what degree *immunologic and other systemic reactions induced by vasectomy may contribute to subsequent aspermatogenesis*. The following observations are pertinent:

1. Rümke and Hellinga (30) reported that a significant number of sterile men with high titers of sperm agglutinins gave a history of injury, infection, or ligation of the vas deferens or epididymis. It was postulated that such obstruction favored sperm extravasation, which then elicited an auto-immune response.

2. In 50 men who underwent ligation of the vas deferens, Phadke and Padukone (31) found a 32 per cent incidence of sperm agglutinins. After surgical correction of the obstruction, positive titers were still demonstrable in 6 of the men.

3. The probable development of auto-immunity to human sperm is similarly inferred from the experience of Schmidt (32) that sterility frequently persists after attempts to reverse a previous vasectomy by inserting a splint made of polyethylene or other tubing.

4. Chiang and Cheng (33) made the following observations concerning the effects of vasectomy performed in rabbits twelve weeks previously: (a) increased body weight; (b) increased weight of the liver, kidney and

spleen; (c) decreased weight of the testes, adrenal glands and prostate; and (d) inhibition of spermatogenesis in a third of the animals.

5. Freund and associates (26) noted varying degrees of aspermatogenesis in 19 of 29 rats after repeated intracutaneous injections of testicular-adjuvant suspensions, but not of liver or kidney suspensions. Such immunologic injury selects the germinal cells. The lesions are usually not associated with inflammation in the intertubular spaces, or with involvement of the Leydig cells, seminal vesicles and prostate. The lack of conspicuous inflammatory changes—comparable to those found in experimental disseminated meningo-encephalomyelitis—might be variously explained by the topographic relationship of the germinal cells to blood vessels, the epididymal elimination of injured cells, and decompensation by enzymes other than those of inflammatory cells.

6. Phadke (34) studied the fate of spermatozoa in patients with obstructive azoospermia and after ligation of the vas deferens. Phagocytosis (largely an intraluminal process) was the chief mechanism involved in the disposal of dead spermatozoa. The spermiophage cells appeared to be derived from the basal layer of cells lining the epididymal tubules. In some instances, such phagocytic activity also occurred in the columnar epithelial lining of the epididymal tubules. Phadke commented: "It is likely that during this process some antigenic components of spermatozoa are also absorbed and transferred to the basal capillaries. This mechanism may be responsible for the development of autoantibodies against spermatozoa in the blood sera of such individuals."

7. Another mechanism for interference by immunologic factors with the metabolism of sperm is suggested by the lowered anaerobic glycolysis of sperm from men with A or AB secretor phenotypes in anti-A or anti-B antisera (35). It is also of interest that Hollinger and Davis (36) demonstrated a marked increase in protein labeling from radioactive glucose by the cryptorchid rat testis, and impairment of glucose catabolism into acid-soluble intermediary metabolites by testicular tissue after the induction of cryptorchidism.

Even *the pathogenesis of postvasectomy psychiatric phenomena* may require modification in the light of these systemic sequelae to vasectomy. Admittedly, considerable psychologic conflict can be precipitated by an ill-advised vasectomy in emotionally disturbed men who have been coerced by wives and their physicians into submitting to the procedure. Many psychiatric explanations have been advanced to explain these psychologic aberrations, including the ensuing threat or challenge to a man's sense of masculinity, "dissonance reduction" (37), and his being "shamed into a resentful acquiescence" (8). The apparent frequency of emotional complications after vasectomy, however, warrants further clarification. For example, Johnson (8) reported that 11 of 83 vasectomized men studied in his psychiatric clinic had been admitted to a psychiatric hospital within one year after operation. Similarly, Ziegler and associates (37) in a study of the effect of vasectomy on psychologic functioning in 22 couples, were impressed by the striking adverse changes and reduced marital satisfaction in husband and wife—as compared with similarly studied couples using birth-control pills—even though there was general satisfaction with the procedure itself. A comparable "weakened sexual desire" was observed in 53 per cent of 1191 men who underwent vasectomy in one clinic in India, even though 92 per cent were "favorable to vasectomy" (38).

Prominent among the metabolic and immunologic factors which could contribute to diminished sexual function and altered nervous-system behavior in such men are the *ravages of diabetogenic hyperinsulinism on the central, peripheral and autonomic nervous system*. In fact, most of the patients in our series complained of narcolepsy, migraine and spontaneous leg cramps—symptoms commonly due to severe reactive hypoglycemia (3–5, 39–41). The development of multiple sclerosis shortly after vasectomy in Case 6 assumes increased significance in view of the following considerations: (a) diabetogenic hyperinsulinism may be a major factor in the pathogenesis of multiple sclerosis (39); and (b) the hyperinsulinized state can be potentiated by testosterone (42), which undoubtedly is released into the testicular tissues— and from there into the systemic circulation—in abnormal amounts following vasectomy. It has been further demonstrated by many investigators that diabetics generally elaborate excessive amounts of biologically-active insulin. There are numerous evidences of the antigenicity of excessive insulin, including (a) synalbumin antagonism in the adult diabetic (43), (b) eosinophilic inflammatory islet infiltrates in the newborn infants of diabetic mothers and in children with acute diabetes, and (c) the simulation of these infiltrates in diabetes induced in rabbits with beef insulin (44) and in rats with guinea pig anti-insulin serum (45). Owing to the frequency of the diabetic-hyperinsulinized state in Jews, it is pertinent that the 2 men with sperm antibody titers of 1:80 and 1:20 reported by Wilson were of Jewish descent (22).

It also has been shown that anaphylactoid and anaphylactic reactions, delayed-type hypersensitivity, and reactivity to a wide variety of pharmacologic and physical stressors can be potentiated by hypoglycemia due to different causes such as fasting, insulin, beta-adrenergic blocking drugs, pertussis vaccine, or adrenalectomy (46, 47). The high ribose content of seminal fluid nucleotides also may be contributory. Goetz and associates (48), studying the effects of ribose on insulin secretion, observed that: (a) the intraportal infusion of D-ribose produces a prompt and sharp increase in pancreatic-vein insulin output; (b) ribose administered intravenously leads to a more striking increase in peripheral insulin concentrations than does ribose administered orally, but without any concomitant rise in the blood glucose concentration; (c) ribose can result in hypoglycemia even when the pancreas is denervated, suggesting that a humoral factor is operative; and (d) the first effect of ribose on insulin output is exerted at a site other than the pancreatic beta cell—presumably in the liver. Beaconsfield and Ginsburg (49) demonstrated a similar hypoglycemic response in both healthy adults and diabetics following the oral ingestion of D-ribose (1 gram per kilogram of body weight); they attributed this reaction to probable increased release of insulin.

Other biologic and immunologic mechanisms influencing cerebral function may be operative in the postvasectomy state. The following observations are pertinent: (a) the recovery of biologically active ribonucleic acid from rat brain after intraperitoneal injection (50, 51); (b) the possible reversal of handedness by a similar procedure (52); (c) the model of experimental allergic encephalomyelitis; and (d) the recent studies of Heath and associates (53, 54) relative to a possible immunologic basis for schizophrenia, summarized as follows, "We conclude that the septal-basal caudate region of the brain contains a unique antigen against which antibody can be created and which is capable of combining with neural cell nuclei of the septal-basal caudate region to induce, possibly through impairment of neurohumoral conduction, aberrations in EEGs associated with schizophrenic behavior. Since serum of schizophrenic patients contains globulin (taraxein) with essentially the same characteristics, we postulate that taraxein may be antibody and that schizophrenia may represent an autoimmune disorder" (53).

Great caution should be used in projecting the purported innocuousness of mass vasectomy programs conducted in famine-threatened countries (such as India) onto the inhabitants of relatively affluent countries. There may be marked differences in the immunologic responsiveness to vasectomy by different populations, for nutritional and other ecologic reasons. For example, there is considerable evidence that the diathesis to the hyperinsulinized state is enhanced in the United States by ingestion of large amounts of sugar and abundant calories (42, 55, 56). The metabolic and tumorigenic effects of androgenic action in the hyperinsulinized state also have been detailed previously (42). Furthermore, in the United States the routine mass immunization to multiple diseases and the repeated exposure to various drugs have activated the population's immune and insulinogenic mechanisms to a high degree. In this regard, Gulbenkian and associates (57) reported prolonged elevation of plasma insulin levels following pertussis sensitization.

For the foregoing reasons, physicians also should resist the mounting demographic pressures to limit conception by "turning off sperm" with "contraceptive pills for men" (58), if such pills become available, until the long-term complications in terms of disease and irreversible sterility are clearly understood. Antispermatogenic agents are known to exert severe cytotoxic effects on spermatids and spermatocytes, and to induce marked interstitial-cell hyperplasia (59). These reservations assume even greater proportions in the case of immunologic methods aimed at rendering men immune to their own sperm (58).

REFERENCES

1. Guttmacher, A. F.: Medical, social, and legal justifications for vasectomy, *Issues in Current Med. Practice 1:* 1 (Oct.) 1964.

2. Campbell, A. A.: The incidence of operations that prevent conception, *Am. J. Obst. & Gynec. 89:* 694, 1964.
3. Roberts, H. J.: Afternoon glucose tolerance testing: a key to the pathogenesis, early diagnosis and prognosis of diabetogenic hyperinsulinism, *J. Am. Geriatrics Soc. 12:* 423, 1964.
4. Roberts, H. J.: The syndrome of narcolepsy and diabetogenic ("functional") hyperinsulinism, with special reference to obesity, diabetes, idiopathic edema, cerebral dysrhythmias and multiple sclerosis (200 patients), *J. Am. Geriatrics Soc. 12:* 926, 1964.
5. Roberts, H. J.: The syndrome of narcolepsy and diabetogenic hyperinsulinism in the American Negro: important clinical, social and public health aspects, *J. Am. Geriatrics Soc. 13:* 852, 1965.
6. Surgeon: Voluntary male sterilisation, *Lancet 1:* 42, 1967.
7. Editorial: Sterilization in man, *Brit. M. J. 1:* 1554, 1966.
8. Johnson, M. H.: Enthusiasm for vasectomy obscures contraindications, *Issues in Current Med. Practice 1:* 10 (Oct.) 1964.
9. Annotations: Autoimmunity to inflammatory exudates, *Lancet 1:* 272, 1966.
10. Bridges, J. M.; Dalby, A. M.; Miller, J. H. D., and Weaver, J. A.: An effect of D-glucose on platelet stickiness, *Lancet 1:* 75, 1965.
11. Sandberg, H., et al.: Alterations in fibrinolytic parameters of subjects with diabetes mellitus, *Am. J. M. Sc. 245:* 153, 1963.
12. Mennon, I. S.: Fibrinolytic response to oral glucose (Letter), *Lancet 2:* 392, 1966.
13. Chakrabarti, R.; Hocking, E. D., and Fearnley, G. R.: Fibrinolytic effect of metformin in coronary-artery disease, *Lancet 2:* 256, 1965.
14. Skovborg, F.; Nielsen, A. V.; Schlichtkrull, J., and Ditzel, J.: Blood-viscosity in diabetic patients, *Lancet 1:* 129, 1966.
15. Skovborg, F.; Nielsen, A. V.; Schlichtkrull, J., and Ditzel, J.: Blood-viscosity in diabetic patients (Letter), *Lancet 2:* 805, 1966.
16. Hennes, A. R., and Awai, K.: Studies of incorporation of radioactivity into lipids by human blood. IV. Abnormal incorporation of acetate 1-C-14 into fatty acids by whole blood and platelets from insulin-independent diabetics, *Diabetes 14:* 209, 1965.
17. Vaughan, J. H.: Auto-immune disease: general considerations, *Postgrad. Med. 40:* 117, 1966.
18. Philips, J. H.; Braun, W., and Plescia, O. J.: Antigenicity of bacterial deoxyribonucleic acid, *Nature 181:* 573, 1958.
19. Chandler, D., and Naldandian, R. M.: DNA autosensitivity, *Am. J. M. Sc. 251:* 145, 1966.
20. Levin, M. B., and Pinkus, H.: Autosensitivity to desoxyribonucleic acid (DNA): report of a case with inflammatory skin lesions controlled by chloroquine, *New England J. Med. 264:* 533, 1961.
21. Katch, S.: Immunology, fertility and infertility: a historical survey, *Am. J. Obst. & Gynec. 77:* 946, 1959.
22. Wilson, L.: Sperm agglutinins in human semen and blood, *Proc. Soc. Exper. Biol. & Med. 85:* 652, 1954.
23. Rümke, P.: The presence of sperm antibodies in the serum of two patients with oligozoospermia, *Vox Sang. 4:* 135, 1954.
24. Freund, J.; Thompson, G. E., and Lipton, M. M.: Aspermatogenesis, anaphylaxis, and cutaneous sensitization induced in the guinea pig by homologous testicular extract, *J. Exper. Med. 101:* 591, 1955.
25. Freund, J.; Lipton, M. M., and Thompson, G. E.: Aspermatogenesis in the guinea pig induced by testicular tissue and adjuvants, *J. Exper. Med. 97:* 711, 1952.
26. Freund, J.; Lipton, M. M., and Thompson, G. E.: Impairment of spermatogenesis in the rat after cutaneous injection of testicular suspension with complete adjuvants, *Proc. Soc. Exper. Biol. & Med. 87:* 408, 1954.

142

27. Mancini, R. E.; Drader, J. A.; Saraceni, D.; Bachmann, A. E.; Lavieri, J. C., and Nemirovski, M.: Immunological and testicular response in man sensitized with human testicular homogenate, *J. Clin. Endocrinol. & Metab. 25:* 859, 1965.

28. Riera, C.; Yantorno, C., and Schulman, S.: Antigenic specificity of seminal plasma and the formation of autoantibodies, *Fed. Proc. 26:* 532, 1967.

29. Yachnin, S.: Studies on the antigenicity of natural and synthetic polynucleotides (Abstract), *J. Clin. Invest. 41:* 1414, 1962.

30. Rümke, P., and Hellinga, G.: Autoantibodies against spermatozoa in sterile men, *Am. J. Clin. Path. 32:* 367, 1959.

31. Phadke, A. M., and Padukone, K.: Presence and significance of autoantibodies against spermatozoa in the blood of men with obstructed vas deferens, *J. Reprod. Fertil. 7:* 163, 1964.

32. Schmidt, S. S.: Cited in *Medical World News,* May 12, 1967, p. 34.

33. Chiang, C., and Cheng, Y.: Histological researches on influence of vasectomy, *J. Formosa M. A. 62:* 47, 1963.

34. Phadke, A. M.: Fate of spermatozoa in cases of obstructive azoospermia and after ligation of vas deferens in man, *J. Reprod. Fertil. 7:* 1, 1964.

35. Ackerman, D. R.: Antibodies of the ABO system and the metabolism of human spermatozoa, *Nature 213:* 253, 1967.

36. Hollinger, M. A., and Davis, J. R.: Metabolic fate of D-glucose-1-C^{14} in slices of scrotal and cryptorchid rat testes, *Fed. Proc. 25:* 313, 1966.

37. Ziegler, F. J.; Rodgers, D. A., and Kriegsman, S. A.: Effect of vasectomy on psychological functioning, *Psychosom. Med. 28:* 50, 1966.

38. Dandekar, K.: After-effects of vasectomy, *Artha Vijnana* (Gokhale Institute of Politics and Economics, Poona, India) *5:* 212, 1963.

39. Roberts, H. J.: An inquiry into the pathogenesis, rational treatment and prevention of multiple sclerosis, with emphasis upon the combined role of diabetogenic hyperinsulinism and recurrent edema, *J. Am. Geriatrics Soc. 14:* 586, 1966.

40. Roberts, H. J.: Spontaneous leg cramps and "restless legs" due to diabetogenic hyperinsulinism: observations on 131 patients, *J. Am. Geriatrics Soc. 13:* 602, 1965.

41. Roberts, H. J.: Chronic refractory fatigue—An "organic" perspective: with emphasis upon the syndrome of narcolepsy and diabetogenic hyperinsulinism, *Med. Times 92:* 1144, 1964.

42. Roberts, H. J.: The role of diabetogenic hyperinsulinism in the pathogenesis of prostatic hyperplasia and malignancy, *J. Am. Geriatrics Soc. 14:* 795, 1966.

43. Vallance-Owen, J.: Synalbumin insulin antagonism, *Diabetes 13:* 241, 1964.

44. Toreson, W. E.; Feldman, R.; Lee, J. C., and Grodsky, G. M.: Pathology of diabetes mellitus produced in rabbits by means of immunization with beef insulin (Abstract), *Am. J. Clin. Path. 42:* 531, 1964.

45. Lacy, P. E., and Wright, P. H.: Allergic interstitial pancreatitis in rats injected with guinea pig anti-insulin serum, *Diabetes 14:* 634, 1965.

46. Adamkiewicz, V. W.: Glycemia and immune responses, *Canad. M. A. J. 88:* 806, 1963.

47. Pieroni, R. E., and Levine, L.: Role of the glycemic state in reactivity to stress, *Fed. Proc. 26:* 802, 1967.

48. Goetz, F. C.; Maney, J. W., and Zaske, R.: Regulation of insulin secretion: the ribose-responsive site (Abstract), *Diabetes 16:* 511, 1967.

49. Beaconsfield, P., and Ginsburg, J.: Hypoglycemia after oral ribose (Letter), *Lancet 2:* 153, 1967.

50. Babich, F. R.; Jacobson, A. L.; Bubash, S., and Jacobson, A.: Transfer of a response to naive rats by injection of ribonucleic acid extracted from trained rats, *Science 149:* 656, 1965.

51. Dennis, M. T. B.: Recovery of biologically active viral ribonucleic acid from rat brain after intraperitoneal injection, *J. Florida M. A. 54:* 465, 1967.

52. Hyden, H., and Egyhazi, E.: Reversal of handedness in rats, *Proc. Nat. Acad. Sc. 49:* 618, 1963.

53. Heath, R. G., and Krupp, I. M.: Schizophrenia as an immunologic disorder. I. Demonstration of antibrain globulins by fluorescent antibody techniques, *Arch. Gen. Psychiat. 16:* 1, 1967.

54. Heath, R. G.; Krupp, I. M.; Byers, L. W., and Liljekvist, J. I.: Schizophrenia as an immunologic disorder. II. Effects of serum protein fractions on brain function, *Arch. Gen. Psychiat. 16:* 10, 1967.

55. Antar, M. A.; Ohlson, M. A., and Hodges, R. E.: Changes in retail market food supplies in the United States in the last seventy years in relation to the incidence of coronary heart disease, with special reference to dietary carbohydrates and essential fatty acids, *Am. J. Clin. Nutrition 14:* 169, 1964.

56. United States Dept. of Agriculture: Supplement for 1961 to "Consumption of Food in the U.S. 1909–52," September 1962 (Table 95).

57. Gulbenkian, A.; Schobert, L.; Nixon, C., and Tabachnick, I. I. A.: Prolonged elevation of plasma insulin levels induced by pertussis sensitization (PS) and concomitant metabolic alterations (Abstract), *Diabetes 16:* 513, 1967.

58. Culliton, B. J.: Turning off sperm, *Sc. News 92:* 452, 1967.

59. Reddy, K. J., and Svoboda, D. J.: Alterations in rat testes due to an antispermatogenic agent: light and electron microscopic study, *Arch. Path. 84:* 376, 1967.

144

A STATISTICAL STUDY OF UNILATERAL PROPHYLACTIC VASECTOMY IN THE PREVENTION OF EPIDIDYMITIS: 1029 CASES

J. ROBERT RINKER, CARL V. HANCOCK AND WILLIAM D. HENDERSON

The prophylactic value of vasectomy in preventing epididymitis associated with urological procedures and retention catheters has been debated.[1] One objection raised was that previous series of cases were not large enough to be statistically significant, which prompted our study.

A conventional vasectomy was done on one side and the other side was used as a control. The first study consisted of 500 men and a second study consisted of 529 men, making a total of 1,029 patients for analysis (table 1).

TABLE 1. *Summary of cases*

	Group 1	Group 2	Total
No. patients	500	529	1029
Epididymitis on non-vasectomized side	23	20	43
Epididymitis on vasectomized side within 7 days	2	0	2
Epididymitis on vasectomized side after 4 years	1	1	2
Funiculitis descending down vas to level of vasectomy	1	1	2

TABLE 2. *Complications*

	Group 1	Group 2	Total
Hematoma at site of vasectomy	2	4	6
Local wound infection (all mild)	2	1	3
			9

The 2 patients in whom epididymitis developed on the vasectomized side 4 years after the procedure had been done are described herein.

Case 1. A 56-year-old man had a stricture of the urethra and prostatic obstruction. Following left vasectomy, cystoscopy and a suprapubic prostatectomy were done without complications. The patient continued to come to the clinic for dilation of the stricture. Four years after vasectomy epididymitis was noted on the left side.

Case 2. A 62-year-old man with residual urine had a vasectomy on the right side only; an additional operation was not done because of other medical problems. The patient returned to the clinic for periodic evaluation of residual urine. Five years later epididymitis developed on the right side but subsided with usual treatment.

Epididymitis in these 2 patients with late occurrence could have been due to hematogenesis or lymphatic spread, recanalization might have taken place or the vas deferens could have been missed at operation. It has been our policy to have tissue reports of the removed section of vas deferens but no report could be found on these 2 patients.

All complications were minor (table 2). One patient was taking cortisone for an eye infection and this was believed to have contributed to the wound infection.

CONCLUSIONS

Since one side was protected by vasectomy in all patients in our series it can be presumed that without vasectomy the incidence of epididymitis could have been twice that which occurred, that is group 1 would have been 46 cases (9.2 per cent) and group 2 would have been 40 cases (7.4 per cent) with a mean of 8.3 per cent for the 1,029 patients.

Since the results of group 1 paralleled so closely those of group 2, a study of 500 patients is statistically significant. The occasional case of epididymitis occurring within a few days after vasectomy can be presumed to have been seeded before the vasectomy was performed. The earlier vasectomy is done, the more effective it will be in preventing epididymitis. If bilateral vasectomy is done before instrumentation or the insertion of a retention catheter, complicating epididymitis should rarely occur.

[1] Graham, J. B. and Grayhack, J. T.: Epididymitis following unilateral vasectomy and prostatic surgery. J. Urol., **87**: 582, 1962.

SUBCUTANEOUS INGUINAL VASECTOMY IN CONJUNCTION WITH ABDOMINAL PROSTATECTOMY

BENJAMIN L. PAGOVICH, MARCEL I. HOROWITZ AND SIDNEY R. WEINBERG

The incidence of epididymitis following prostatic surgery varies from 10 to 15 per cent.[1,2] Epididymitis is a serious complication, often accounting for a greater morbidity than the actual prostatectomy. Therefore, it is generally accepted that prophylactic vasectomy has more benefits than disadvantages, as the incidence of

is that this procedure carries its own complications such as vasitis, hematoma and abscess formation.

The technique to be presented obviates the complications of scrotal surgery and allows for prophylactic bilateral vasectomy to be incidental to prostatectomy.

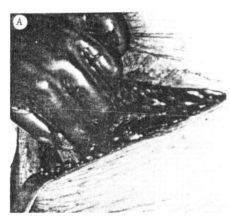 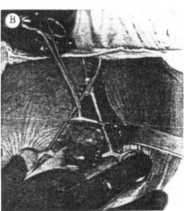

A, spermatic cord grasped at external inguinal ring. *B*, vasectomy done on isolated vas deferens

epididymitis in association with prostatectomy in patients with vasectomy has been as low as 5 to 6 per cent. However, because of complications the value of routine scrotal vasectomy for prevention of epididymitis has been debatable. The argument against routine prophylactic vasectomy

PROCEDURE

Subcutaneous inguinal vasectomy has been done in conjunction with abdominal prostatic enucleation. A suprapubic transverse incision was used in most cases. In 8 patients a longitudinal midline incision was used, either when a previous transverse suprapubic incision had been present or when the patient was an extremely poor surgical risk so that the small amount of time saved in closing the vertical incision was deemed important by the operator.

The vasectomy was done after exposure of the rectus fascia and prior to prostatic enucleation to avoid retrograde infection. The spine of the pubis was identified and by blunt dissection, using the thumb and index fingers, the cord

[1] Schmidt, S. S. and Hinman, F.: The effect of vasectomy upon the incidence of epididymitis after prostatectomy: an analysis of 810 operations. J. Urol., 63: 872–881, 1950.

[2] Haralambidis, G. and Spinelli, A. N.: Vasectomy: an evaluation. J. Urol., 89: 591–594, 1963.

146

structures were isolated below the external ring and brought into view (part *A* of figure). The vas was easily detected and grasped with a clamp. The fibrous sheath of the vas was incised and the vas was delivered from its envelope, clamped and cut with either a Bovie knife or a scalpel. The 2 ends were either ligated with chromic catgut or fulgurated (part *B* of figure). The cord was replaced in its normal position. The same procedure was carried out on the opposite side.

This procedure has been done successfully in 93 cases from 1965 to 1967. Epididymitis has not occurred postoperatively. Postoperative urinary antiseptics were given to 89 of the 93 patients.

SUMMARY

The advantages of subcutaneous bilateral vasectomy are: 1) it is performed through the same incision that is used for prostatectomy, 2) manipulation of the scrotum is avoided and 3) it saves operative time.

Hormonal Physiology of Vasectomy

PITUITARY GONADOTROPHINS (FOLLICLE-STIMULATING HORMONE AND INTERSTITIAL CELL-STIMULATING HORMONE) AND SEMINAL VESICULAR FRUCTOSE AFTER LONG-TERM VASECTOMY IN BULLS

A. M. RAKHA, Ph.D., and G. IGBOELI, Ph.D.

Current interest in vasectomy as a method of sterilization requires a thorough investigation of its after effects. In a previous report[1] it was suggested that the reduced rate of sperm flow in the epididymis of chronically vasectomized bulls may by some unknown mechanism decrease the rate of spermatogenesis. The possibility of an integrating factor regulating spermatogenesis, epididymal sperm flow, storage, and resorption has also been suggested.[2] Whether this regulation is hormonal, neural, or physical is not clear, and it is intended by this study to investigate the possible role of gonadotrophins in this process.

The pituitary glands and seminal vesicles were collected from five chronically vasectomized (1–5 years vasectomy), and four comparable intact bulls soon after slaughter.

Each pituitary was trimmed, weighed, and the anterior lobe was frozen on Dry Ice, then freeze-dried (FD), ground to a fine powder, and stored in a desicator. The follicle-stimulating hormone (FSH) and interstitial cell-stimulating hormone (ICSH) determinations were run as single assays (2 + 1 design) on Sprague-Dawley female rats and the potency of the preparations were calculated.[3] FSH was determined by the augmentation method;[4] four animals were used per group, and each received 20 I.U. of human chorionic gonadotrophin (HCG). The standard doses used were 0.1 and 0.2 mg. of NIH-FSH-P1; saline extracts of 35–50 mg. of pituitary powder represented the unknown. The total dose was 3 ml. (6 × 0.5 ml.). ICSH was determined by the ovarian ascorbic acid depletion method.[5] The standard doses used were 2 μg. and 4 μg. of NIH-LH-B6; a saline extract of 0.6 mg. of pituitary powder represented the unknown. Four animals were used per group. All preparations were given as a single intraperitoneal injection (0.5 ml.) and the animals killed 4 hr. later, both ovaries bulked, and the ascorbic acid concentration determined.[6,7] The degree of depletion was estimated by reference to the mean value of a control group.

The fructose concentrations of the seminal vesicles were determined.[8]

The present results showed no differences in the pituitary FSH and ICSH concentrations or content between intact and vasectomized bulls.

In their previous report, Igboeli and Rakha observed that chronic vasectomy resulted in a slight reduction in the rate of spermatogenesis. Although the present findings would tend to rule out hormonal intervention in this process, the possibility of an alteration in the relationship between the rates of ICSH and FSH synthesis and/or release, or an alteration in the response of the testes following vasectomy cannot be overlooked. However, when androgen production of the testes was assessed by the concentration of fructose in the seminal vesicles, no differences were observed. This is in agreement with previous findings of Skinner and Rowson.[9] In addition how-

TABLE 1. *Pituitary FSH and ICSH Levels and Seminal Vesicular Fructose in Vasectomized Animals*

Group	SV* fructose	FSH activity in terms of NIH-FSH-S₁			ICSH activity in terms of NIH-LH-S₁			Ratio ICSH/FSH
		Concentration (FD)	Content	λ	Concentration (FD)	Content	λ	
	mg./100 gm.	μg./mg.	μg.		μg./mg.	μg.		
Intact	222	1.66(0.53–3.15)	843.3	0.10	28.52(2.85–61.60)	14488.2	0.23	17.18
	233	1.60(0.36–3.35)	580.8	0.12	17.92(10.70–27.18)	6505.0	0.29	11.20
	233	1.63(0.96–3.02)	255.9	0.17	10.94(3.50–13.3)	1717.6	0.24	6.71
	256	1.20(0.24–2.16)	229.2	0.17	8.88(0.96–9.79)	1696.1	0.22	7.40
Mean ± S.E.	236 ± 7.2	1.52 ± 0.11	477.3 ± 145.80		16.57 ± 4.43	6101.7 ± 301.60		10.90
Vasecto-mized	330	1.89(0.61–2.89)	1032	0.25	7.85(3.75–11.68)	4286	0.30	4.15
	259	0.87(0.06–0.88)	724	0.15	6.38(1.6–7.29)	5308	0.19	7.33
	181	1.06(0.08–1.39)	524	0.16	9.95(2.71–10.45)	4915	0.22	9.39
	256	1.94(0.80–3.98)	565	0.11	21.27(7.36–35.35)	6190	0.28	10.96
		1.66(0.67–3.65)	354	0.10	30.39(7.01–69.90)	5045	0.22	18.31
Mean ± S.E.	256.5 ± 30.4	1.48 ± 0.22	640 ± 114.40		15.17 ± 4.62	5149 ± 309.75		10.25

* SV refers to the concentration of fructose/100 gm. of the seminal vesicles.

ever, these authors reported a significant reduction in the fructose and citric acid content of the ampullae of vasectomized pubescent animals, which was attributed to a purely physical interruption of the normal passage of testosterone along the vas deferens.

Further work is required to investigate the physical and neural factors which may result from vasectomy and which may operate to alter the normal equilibrium between spermatogenesis, sperm flow, and sperm resorption.

SUMMARY

The concentrations and contents of pituitary gonadotrophins (FSH and ICSH) and seminal vesicular fructose, in five chronically vasectomized (1–5 years vasectomy) and four intact bulls, were determined.

The present results showed that vasectomy in bulls did not alter the pituitary FSH or ICSH concentration and content. Similarly, there was no effect on androgen production of the testes as expressed in terms of fructose concentration in the seminal vesicles.

Acknowledgments. The authors are grateful to D. K. Dutta-Roy for his advice in the statistical analysis; Messrs. D. Lungu, J. Parshotam, and S. Chilinda for technical assistance; and to the Endocrine Study Section of the National Institutes of Health for the standard pituitary hormone preparations.

REFERENCES

1. IGBOELI, G., AND RAKHA, A. M. Bull testicular and epididymal functions after long-term vasectomy. *J Anim Sci 31:*72, 1970.
2. AMANN, R. P., AND ALMQUIST, J. O. Reproductive capacity of dairy bulls: VI. Effect of unilateral vasectomy and ejaculation on sperm reserves; aspects of epididymal physiology. *J Reprod Fertil 3:*260, 1962.
3. GADDUM, J. H. Simplified mathematics for bioassays. *J Pharm Pharmacol 5:*345, 1953.
4. STEELMAN, S. L., AND POHLEY, F. M. Assay of follicle stimulating hormone based on the augmentation with HCG. *Endocrinology 53:*604, 1953.
5. PARLOW, A. F. "Bioassay of pituitary luteinizing hormone by depletion of ovarian ascorbic acid." In *Human Pituitary Gonadotrophins,* Albert, A. Ed. Thomas, Springfield, Ill. 1961, pp. 300–310.
6. MAIKEL, R. P. A rapid procedure for the determination of adrenal ascorbic acid. Application of the Sullivan and Clarks method to tissue analysis. *Analyt Biochem 1:*498, 1960.
7. ROBERTSON, H. A., AND RAKHA, A. M. The se-

quence, time and duration, of the release of follicle stimulating hormone and luteinizing hormone in relation to oestrus and ovulation in the sheep. *J Endocr* 35:177, 1966.

8. LINDNER, H. R., AND MANN, T. Relationship between the content of androgenic steroids in the testes and the secretory activity of the seminal vesicles in the bull. *J Endocr* 21:241, 1960.

9. SKINNER, J. D., AND ROWSON, L. E. A. Some effects of unilateral cryptorchism and vasectomy on sexual development of the pubescent ram and bull. *J. Endocr.* 42:311, 1968.

Adrenergic Innervation of the Male Reproductive Ducts in Some Mammals. II. Effects of Vasectomy and Castration

K.-A. Norberg, Paul L. Risley
and U. Ungerstedt

The normal distribution of adrenergic nerves to vasa deferentia of various species was observed by several authors[1-4] using a highly specific fluorescence histochemical method[5-7]. Cell bodies of adrenergic neurons in ganglia near the prostatic end of the vas deferens synapse with preganglionic fibres of the hypogastric nerves[2,4,8], and give rise to adrenergic axons of the vas deferens and adjacent organs[9-11]. The present authors[12] recently surveyed the testis and its associated ducts in several mammals with the aim of determining differences in distributions of adrenergic neurons in various regions. This study was undertaken to obtain experimental evidence concerning the course of the adrenergic innervation, and to determine if alterations might result from castration and reduced male sex hormone activity.

Histochemical procedures used were referred to previously[12], and followed the routine technique of this laboratory for noradrenaline (NA) localization by fluorescence microscopy[2,13,14]. 6 Sprague-Dawley albino rats (160–200 g) were uni- or bilaterally vasectomized by removing a one cm section of the duct. In unilateral cases, opposite unoperated ducts served as normal controls. Comparisons also were made with unoperated specimens. In bilateral operations, one vas deferens was completely sectioned, but blood vessels along the anterior margin were not disturbed on the opposite side. Tissues were obtained from the remaining ends of the operated ducts at 2, 6 and 14 days after operation, but 1 rat was retained for 6 months. One unilaterally vasectomized cat was sacrificed after 6 days.

On the epididymal side of the site of vasectomy, fluorescent adrenergic terminals, normally present, were not evident in the cauda epididymidis, indicating that the reactive NA disappears from the axons in 2–3 days (compare Figures 1 and 2). When blood vessels along the anterior border were not removed, adrenergic terminals were observed in the anterior muscle wall of the vas deferens, but were absent mainly from its posterior wall and the cauda epididymidis. Muscular atrophy was not apparent even after long-term vasectomy (6 months), but,

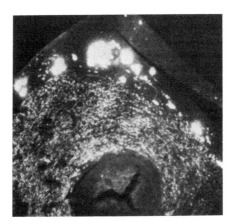

Fig. 1. Vas deferens, rat, from the prostatic side after vasectomy. Varicose terminals in musculature appear normal but accumulation of fluorescent material is extensive in the non-terminal nerve trunks. × 45.

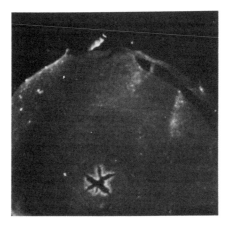

Fig. 2. Vas deferens, rat, from the epididymal side after vasectomy. Complete absence of fluorescent terminals and trunks. All white spots in photograph are artifacts. × 45.

154

in this case, the existence of widely separated, less frequent, and uniformly distributed terminals suggested reinnervation from the severed axons at the prostatic end.

On the prostatic sides of sectioned vasa deferentia no alterations of the adrenergic terminals or their varicosities were apparent. However, a striking increase of fluorescence intensity was observed in the non-terminal nerve trunks in this region, indicating an accumulation of reactive substances in the axons[14,15].

Ten adult rats were castrated totally and sacrificed 30, 60 and 180 days later. The effects were associated with the general reduction in size of epididymides and vasa

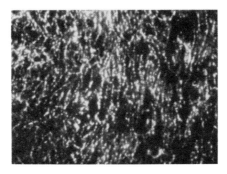

Fig. 3. Vas deferens, normal adult rat, showing typical varicose adrenergic terminal plexus in smooth muscle. Compare with Figure 4. × 210.

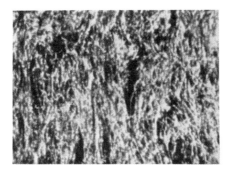

Fig. 4. Vas deferens, castrate rat. Abundant numbers of terminals occur, often superimposed upon each other because of muscle atrophy. Note smaller varicosities. Compare with Figure 3. × 210.

deferentia. Normally, adrenergic terminals are distributed in smooth muscle walls of the vas deferens and cauda epididymidis. Before castration, adrenergic terminals penetrate the muscle walls of epididymal ducts, but afterwards, they are located mainly along the outer margins of the muscle layer, as they normally appear in blood vessels. In the vas deferens, the reduced thickness of the muscle wall results in a much closer and more dense adrenergic ground plexus. Terminals are thrown into slight folds, and varicosities seemed less sharply defined, smaller, and more difficult to identify (Figures 3 and 4). Background fluorescence also was somewhat increased in castrates. While these differences in appearance might result from technical errors, the observed effects were consistent and appear to reflect altered tissue states after castration.

The occurrence of synapses between the hypogastric nerves and the adrenergic neurons innervating the vas deferens has been demonstrated by the failure of denervation after hypogastric nerve section[8,11]. The present results provide the further positive evidence that sectioning of the vas deferens results in the disappearance of the green fluorescent materials from the terminal axons on the post-ganglionic side of the lesion. In the cat, however, adrenergic nerves to the ductuli efferentes and caput epididymidis[12] remained present after vasectomy, but the plexus to the cauda epididymidis and epididymal vas deferens was not visible. Adrenergic nerves evidently reach the caput epididymidis by way of the superior spermatic nerve from the lumbar sympathetics in this species.

After castration, the adrenergic plexus was distributed to the smooth muscle in a manner that recalled the distribution of the cholinesterase reactive plexus of the rat epididymis[16,17]. In the cauda epididymidis, it appeared also to be confined mainly to the peripheral surface of the duct walls. In normal animals this is true for the more weakly innervated ducts of the upper cauda and lower corpus epididymidis. The effect was more readily apparent in the ChE-positive plexus than in the adrenergic one, where no clear reduction in fluorescence intensity could be recognized in individual axons. Absence of male sex hormones has only slight effects on the morphology of the adrenergic nerves to the male reproductive ducts, attributable mainly to the simultaneous atrophy of smooth muscle elements and associated tissue changes[18].

156

[1] B. Falck, Acta physiol. scand. *56*, Suppl. 197 (1962).

[2] K.-A. Norberg and B. Hamberger, Acta physiol. scand. *63*, Suppl. 238 (1964).

[3] B. Falck, Ch. Owman and N. O. Sjöstrand, Experientia *21*, 98 (1965).

[4] Ch. Owman and N. O. Sjöstrand, Z. Zellforsch. *66*, 300 (1965).

[5] B. Falck, N.-Å. Hillarp, G. Thieme and A. Torp, J. Histochem. Cytochem. *10*, 348 (1962).

[6] H. Corrodi and N.-Å. Hillarp, Helv. chim. Acta *46*, 2425 (1963).

[7] H. Corrodi and N.-Å. Hillarp, Helv. chim. Acta *47*, 911 (1964).

[8] D. Jacobowitz and G. B. Koelle, J. Pharmac. exp. Ther. *148*, 225 (1965).

[9] N. O. Sjöstrand, Acta physiol. scand. *54*, 306 (1962a).

[10] N. O. Sjöstrand, Acta physiol. scand. *56*, 376 (1962b).

[11] N. O. Sjöstrand, Acta physiol. scand. *65*, Suppl. 257 (1965).

[12] K.-A. Norberg, P. L. Risley and U. Ungerstedt, Z. Zellforsch. *76*, 278 (1967).

[13] B. Falck and Ch. Owman, Acta Univ. Lund, II, 7, 1 (1965).

[14] A. Dahlström and K. Fuxe, Z. Zellforsch. *62*, 602 (1964).

[15] A. Dahlström, J. Anat. *99*, 677 (1965).

[16] P. L. Risley and C. N. Skrepetos, Anat. Rec. *148*, 231 (1964a).

[17] P. L. Risley and C. N. Skrepetos, Anat. Rec. *150*, 195 (1964b).

[18] Acknowledgments: This work was supported in part by a research grant (No. B66-257) from the Swedish Medical Research Council. The second author was on leave from the Biology Department, University of Oregon, Eugene (Oregon, USA) aided by a special Research Fellowship granted by the National Council for Child Health and Human Development, National Institute of Health, USA Dept. of Health, Education and Welfare. Use of facilities of the Department of Physiology I of the Karolinska Institute with the permission of Prof. U. S. von Euler and Research Docent R. Eliasson is greatly appreciated. For skillful technical assistance, we are grateful to Mrs. Ulla Flyger and Miss Berith Hanson.

SOME EFFECTS OF UNILATERAL CRYPTORCHISM AND VASECTOMY ON SEXUAL DEVELOPMENT OF THE PUBESCENT RAM AND BULL

J. D. SKINNER AND L. E. A. ROWSON

INTRODUCTION

Hitherto, the effect of experimental cryptorchism on the endocrine function of the testes has been studied mainly in laboratory animals. Some authors have suggested that it produces hypertrophy of the testicular interstitium (Bouin & Ancel, 1903; Sand, 1921; Clegg, 1961) but Moore (1924b) believed that this hypertrophy was only relative to shrinkage of the seminiferous tubule. Some authors claimed that androgen secretion is unaffected in the crytorchid testis as indicated by the ejaculate volume, or weight and cytological appearance of the accessory glands (Moore & Gallagher, 1930; Jeffries, 1931; Antliff & Young, 1957) but others did not agree because they have found a reduction of accessory gland weight (Nelson, 1937; Moore, 1944), of the radioactive index (Morehead & Morgan, 1967) and of the fructose and citric acid content (Clegg, 1960). They concluded that androgen production is reduced. Urinary androgen excretion (Kimeldorf, 1948; Engberg, 1949) and testicular androgenic enzyme activity (Llaurado & Dominguez, 1963; Kormano, Harkonen & Kontinen, 1964) are also diminished by cryptorchism. In addition, Hanes & Hooker (1937) found, in two pooled samples of porcine cryptorchid testes, only half as much androgen per unit weight as in scrotal testes.

The effect of artificial cryptorchism on spermatogenesis in the mature testis has long been known (Griffiths, 1893) and has been described in great detail by Carl Moore and his co-workers (Moore, 1924a, 1926; Moore & Oslund, 1924; Moore & Quick, 1924a) who, following the original suggestion of Crew (1922), established the thermo-regulatory role of the scrotum.

The object of the present experiments was to examine the effects of unilateral cryptorchism on testicular androgen production, spermatogenesis and development of the reproductive tract of the pubescent ram and bull. The parameters used included the weight and morphology of the tract, testicular hormone content, histology and histochemistry of the testis, ampullae and seminal vesicles, and the concentrations of fructose and citric acid in the ampullae and seminal vesicles. A preliminary report has already been published (Skinner & Rowson, 1967).

MATERIAL AND METHODS

The experimental animals consisted of 20 Suffolk and Suffolk × Welsh Mountain lambs. Five of them were rendered unilaterally cryptorchid for 16 weeks, another five were made unilaterally cryptorchid for 8 weeks only, after which each cryptorchid testis was returned to the scrotum for a further 8 weeks. Another five lambs were made unilaterally cryptorchid for 16 weeks but were vasectomized on the contralateral side, and the remaining five lambs were unilaterally vasectomized only for 16 weeks. Five Friesian calves, one 2-yr.-old Suffolk ram with a naturally occurring unilateral cryptorchism and one 3-yr-old stallion also with a naturally occurring unilateral cryptorchism were also investigated. Artificial unilateral cryptorchism was produced in 15 lambs and four calves by returning the left testis to the abdominal cavity through the inguinal ring, within 2 weeks of birth. In five lambs biopsies were performed on both testes at the time when the cryptorchid testis was returned to the scrotum after 8 weeks. In five lambs vasectomy was performed on the contralateral scrotal side and in five lambs unilateral vasectomy only was performed, within 2 weeks of birth. All the lambs and three calves were killed 16 weeks after the operation. The remaining calf was killed 32 weeks after the operation, and the left testis of a fifth calf was returned to the abdomen at 32 weeks of age for 16 weeks until slaughter.

At autopsy, the reproductive tract was dissected, the testes and accessory glands weighed and the diameter of the ampullae measured. Slices of tissue were removed for histology and the testes, seminal vesicles and ampullae stored in solid carbon dioxide for later assay.

Histological and histochemical techniques

Pieces of testes were fixed in Bouin's fluid or Zenker-formol solution. Pieces of seminal vesicles, ampullae and bulbo-urethral glands were fixed in Bouin's fluid. The

160

Bouin-fixed material was dehydrated in ethanol, cleared in cedarwood oil and embedded in paraffin wax; sections, 6 μ thick, were stained with Delafield's haematoxylin and chromotrope 2R. The tissue fixed in Zenker-formol solution was postchromed in potassium dichromate, washed, dehydrated, cleared, embedded in paraffin wax, sectioned and treated with Sudan black as described by Threadgold (1957) in his method 1.

Further slices of testis were frozen on cryostat chucks with solid CO_2, sections 16 μ thick were cut and incubated for 3 hr. at 37° to demonstrate the presence of Δ^5-3β-hydroxysteroid dehydrogenase activity as described by Hay & Deane (1966) and Mann, Rowson, Short & Skinner (1967). Other sections were incubated for 1 hr. in a medium containing a 0·3 % solution of reduced nicotinamide-adenine dinucleotide phosphate (NADPH; Boehringer) to demonstrate NAD-tetrazolium reductase (diaphorase) as described by Hay & Deane (1966); the reaction must be positive if NAD-dependent enzymes are to be visualized.

The right and left side of each tract was dealt with separately, the scrotal side serving as control, and the results were analysed by means of Student's paired t test after converting to logarithmic values.

Assay of androgens

The concentration of testosterone and androstenedione was determined according to the method described by Mann et al. (1967) and Skinner, Booth, Rowson & Karg (1968).

Assay of fructose and citric acid

The concentrations of fructose and citric acid in the seminal vesicles were estimated according to the method of Lindner & Mann (1960). In the ampullae, which were invariably small, the method of determination was modified as follows: each ampulla was cut longitudinally down the middle into two halves. For fructose: 0·25 g. tissue was finely ground in a mortar with 5 ml. absolute ethanol and 2 ml. distilled water, centrifuged, and the supernatant fluid poured into a flask. The residue was reground with 5 ml. absolute ethanol, centrifuged and the supernatant added to the flask. These combined extracts were evaporated to 2 ml. on a rotary evaporator, and deproteinized with 0·25 ml. satd. $Ba(OH)_2$ and 0·25 ml. 0·17 M-$ZnSO_4$. For citric acid: 0·25 g. tissue from an equivalent part of the other half of the gland was finely ground with 3 ml. 15 % trichloracetic acid and 2 ml. distilled water, centrifuged, and the chemical estimation carried out on the supernatant.

RESULTS

Morphological observations

The appearance of the reproductive tract in lambs with experimental unilateral cryptorchism or vasectomized lambs is illustrated in Plate 1, which shows that the testis, epididymis, vas deferens and ampulla on the cryptorchid side are smaller than those on the contralateral side. The same effect was found in the calves. Where vasectomy was performed on the contralateral scrotal side the epididymis was distended with fluid with a resultant increase in size; there was no apparent difference in size between the ampullae on the vasectomized and cryptorchid side. There was also no apparent difference in the size of the bilateral scrotal testes between the

161

vasectomized and the non-vasectomized sides. Only small differences were apparent between the vasa deferentia and between the ampullae. No differences were found between either the seminal vesicles or the bulbo-urethral glands.

Histological and histochemical findings

The histochemical appearance of the cryptorchid testes is compared with that of the contralateral scrotal testes in Plate 2. There was an apparent increase in the amount of interstitial tissue, while the seminiferous tubules did not enlarge. The cryptorchid testis resembled the prepuberal normal testis (Skinner et al. 1968). There was no evidence of an increase in the number of Leydig cells. On the contrary, a decrease was observed in Δ^5-3β-hydroxysteroid dehydrogenase activity in both the bull and the stallion (Pl. 2, figs. 1, 2) and practically no lipid was seen in the interstitium of the cryptorchid gonad (Pl. 2, figs. 3, 4). An interesting observation in the stallion (Pl. 2, figs. 5, 6) was that NADPH diaphorase activity in the cryptorchid testis was greatest in the tubule, but in the interstitium in the scrotal testis. This phenomenon, however, was not observed in the cryptorchid testis of the pubescent bull (Pl. 2, figs. 7, 8).

In the seminiferous tubules, supporting cells did not differentiate into Sertoli cells, nor was there evidence for the presence of lipid in the supporting cells (Pl. 2, figs. 3, 4). Gonocytes were still present in the testes of lambs that had been cryptorchid for 16 weeks but were missing from the seminiferous tubules of the ram that had been cryptorchid for 2 yr. (Pl. 2, fig. 9). After 8 weeks there appeared to be no spermatogenic activity in the cryptorchid testis, whereas in the contralateral scrotal testis spermatogenesis may just have started (Pl. 2, figs. 12, 13). Eight weeks after the cryptorchid testes had been returned to the scrotum, they showed some signs of spermatogenic activity, although apparently abnormal, and their seminiferous tubules had doubled in diameter; in the contralateral scrotal testis the final stages of spermatogenesis are apparent, and the diameter of the seminiferous tubule had also doubled (Pl. 2, figs. 14, 15).

No histological differences were observed between the two scrotal testes in unilateral vasectomized lambs.

Testicular androgen concentration

The weights of the testes, seminiferous tubule diameters and testicular androgen content are shown in Tables 1 and 2. In the ram (Table 1) the absolute content of androgen, but not its concentration, in the cryptorchid testis was reduced about ten times; the reduction in content could thus be accounted for by the reduced size of the gonad. Some samples of cryptorchid testes had a higher androstenedione concentration, but the results were equivocal. In Table 1 the androgen contents from five scrotal testes in the top group are compared with 12 scrotal testes from normal rams (Skinner et al. 1968). More androgen is present in the unilateral scrotal testis than in the bilateral scrotal gonad. There were only small differences in bilateral scrotal testes when one side was vasectomized.

In the bull androstenedione concentration exceeded testosterone concentration in the cryptorchid testis. This was not the case in the testis that had been cryptorchid for 16 weeks, and was examined at 48 weeks of age. Differences in weight between the cryptorchid testis and scrotal testis were not as great in the bull as in the ram.

Table 1. *Comparison of mean weight, diameter of seminiferous tubules and content of androstenedione (Ad) and testosterone (Te) in testes of unilateral cryptorchid and/or vasectomized rams*

	No.	Weight (g.)	Diameter (μ) of semini-ferous tubules	Ad μg./ 100 g.	Ad μg./ testis	Te μg./ 100 g.	Te μg./ testis	Ad:Te ratio
Unilateral cryptorchid 16 weeks								
Abdominal testis	5	11·0	59·7	5·26	0·579	11·60	1·277	1:2·2
Scrotal testis	5	141·7	192·8	2·94	4·165	10·22	14·470	1:3·5
Unilateral cryptorchid 8 weeks, then returned to scrotum for 8 weeks								
Replaced abdominal testis	5	24·7	94·4 (50·8)*	3·23†	0·798	36·50†	9·016	1:11·3
Scrotal testis	5	72·2	150·2 (75·5)*	5·40†	0·899	28·13†	20·309	1:5·2
Unilateral cryptorchid 2 yr.								
Abdominal testis	1	13·6	66·9	—	—	—	—	—
Scrotal testis	1	169·4	224·4	—	—	—	—	—
Unilateral cryptorchid 16 weeks								
Abdominal testis	5	9·7	59·6	7·56†	0·733	5·60†	0·543	1:0·7
Vasectomized scrotal testis	5	94·2	162·8	4·20†	3·957	6·30†	5·934	1:1·5
Unilaterally vasectomized 16 weeks								
Normal side	5	85·6	151·7	2·40†	2·054	5·90†	5·050	—
Vasectomized side	5	79·9	152·7	1·90†	1·508	6·40†	5·114	—
Bilateral scrotal testes from rams 16–20 weeks of age (from Skinner *et al.* 1968)	12	125·8	178·2	0·55	0·630	7·08	7·270	—

* Diameter at biopsy at 8 weeks.   † Estimated from pooled sample.

Table 2. *Comparison of mean weight, diameter of seminiferous tubules and content of androstenedione (Ad) and testosterone (Te) in testes of unilateral cryptorchid calves*

	No.	Weight (g.)	Diameter (μ) of seminiferous tubules	Ad μg./ 100 g.	Ad μg./ gland	Te μg./ 100 g.	Te μg./ gland	Ad:Te ratio
Unilateral cryptorchid birth, 16 weeks								
Abdominal testis	2	18·4	68·6	17·9	3·294	8·20	1·509	1:0·5
Scrotal testis	2	37·4	123·6	10·80	4·077	59·50	22·250	1:5·5
Unilateral cryptorchid birth, 32 weeks								
Abdominal testis	1	26·1	78·9	—	—	—	—	—
Scrotal testis	1	111·3	214·7	—	—	—	—	—
Unilateral cryptorchid 32–48 weeks								
Abdominal testis	1	26·5	121·8	2·24	0·594	29·10	7·711	1:12·9
Scrotal testis	1	175·0	240·2	4·33	7·578	46·32	81·060	1:10·7

Weights of accessory glands and the concentrations of fructose and citric acid in the seminal vesicles and ampullae

The weight of the epididymides, vasa deferentia, bulbo-urethrals, seminal vesicles and ampullae and the diameter of the latter are shown in Table 3 for rams and Table 4 for calves. The epididymal weights were consistently much greater on the scrotal side as was the weight of the vasa deferentia. The diameter of ampullae in the ram on the cryptorchid side was smaller than that of ampullae on the scrotal side, and they weighed less (Pl. 1). When the contralateral scrotal side was vasectomized this

163

Table 3. *Comparison of mean weight of epididymides, vasa deferentia, bulbo-urethrals, seminal vesicles and ampullae and concentrations of fructose and citric acid in the seminal vesicles and ampullae in unilateral cryptorchid and/or vasectomized rams*

	No.	Epididymis weight (g.)	Vas deferens weight (g.)	Ampulla Weight (g.)	Ampulla Diameter (mm.)	Ampulla Fructose mg./100 g.	Ampulla Fructose mg./gland	Ampulla Citric acid mg./100 g.	Ampulla Citric acid mg./gland	Seminal vesicle Weight (g.)	Seminal vesicle Fructose (mg./100 g.)	Seminal vesicle Citric acid (mg./100 g.)	Bulbo-urethral weight (g.)
Unilateral cryptorchid 16 weeks													
Scrotal side	5	13·4	0·87	1·08	3·96	130	1·413	82	0·895	1·9	165	34	1·00
Abdominal side	5	2·1	0·47	0·85	3·70	94	0·796	64	0·553	1·9	168	35	1·00
Difference		11·3**	0·40**	0·23**	0·24**	36*	0·615**	18*	0·342**	0	−3	−1	0
Unilateral cryptorchid 8 weeks then returned to scrotum for 8 weeks													
Scrotal side	5	9·6	0·77	0·79	3·92	36	0·299	16	0·137	1·5	126	40	0·7
Abdominal side	5	4·9	0·58	0·66	3·86	15	0·135	11	0·063	1·4	127	37	0·6
Difference		4·7**	0·19**	0·13*	0·06	21*	0·164**	5*	0·074**	0·1	−1	3	0·1
Unilateral cryptorchid 2 yr.													
Scrotal side	1	22·5	1·40	1·75	5·22	130	2·315	50	0·875	5·4	346	60	2·7
Abdominal side	1	3·5	0·80	1·25	3·60	83	1·038	30	0·375	5·2	354	70	2·5
Difference		19·0	0·60	0·50	1·62	47	1·277	20	0·500	0·2	−8	−10	0·2
Unilateral vasectomized 16 weeks													
Scrotal side	5	21·2	0·77	0·72	3·80	50	0·366	20	0·166	1·7	123	28	1·1
Unilateral cryptorchid 16 weeks													
Abdominal side	5	2·6	0·45	0·74	3·90	67	0·505	26	0·198	1·7	132	29	1·1
Difference		18·6**	0·32**	−0·02	−0·10	−17*	−0·139**	−6	−0·032	0	−8	−1	0
Unilateral vasectomized 16 weeks													
Normal side	5	12·1	1·00	0·98	3·8	69	0·937	32	0·318	1·57	110	24	0·9
Vasectomized side	5	18·0	0·70	0·80	3·7	63	0·694	28	0·264	1·54	112	27	0·9
Difference		−5·9	0·30	0·18**	0·1	6	0·243**	4	0·054**	0·03	−2	−3	0

* $P < 0.05$. ** $P < 0.01$.

Table 4. *Comparison of mean weight of epididymides, vasa deferentia, bulbo-urethrals, seminal vesicles and ampullae and fructose and citric acid concentrations in the seminal vesicles and ampullae of unilateral cryptorchid calves*

	No.	Epididymis weight (g.)	Vas deferens weight (g.)	Ampulla Weight (g.)	Ampulla Fructose mg./100 g.	Ampulla Fructose mg./gland	Ampulla Citric acid mg./100 g.	Ampulla Citric acid mg./gland	Seminal vesicle Weight (g.)	Seminal vesicle Fructose mg./100 g.	Seminal vesicle Citric acid mg./100 g.	Bulbo-urethral weight (g.)
Unilateral cryptorchid birth 16 weeks												
Scrotal side	3	2·9	0·9	1·36	25	0·374	20	0·311	6·7	80	34	0·7
Abdominal side	3	1·6	0·5	1·3	23	0·301	19	0·244	6·7	87	37	0·7
Difference		1·3	0·4	0·23	2	0·073	1	0·007	0	−7	−3	0
Unilateral cryptorchid birth 32 weeks												
Scrotal side	1	7·4	1·1	3·60	90	0·324	120	0·367	14·8	210	145	2·6
Abdominal side	1	3·1	0·8	3·30	74	0·244	90	0·297	14·3	220	150	2·5
Difference		4·3	0·3	0·30	16	0·080	30	0·070	0·5	−10	−5	0·1
Unilateral cryptorchid 32–48 weeks												
Scrotal side	1	15·7	2·5	6·90	94	6·486	75	5·275	34·0	290	160	3·9
Abdominal side	1	6·0	2·5	6·20	50	3·100	40	2·480	32·0	294	150	3·9
Difference		9·7	0	0·70	44	3·386	35	2·795	2·0	14	10	0

164

difference disappeared. Cytological differences between the two ampullae were very small, but the content of fructose and citric acid of the non-vasectomized scrotal ampullae were much greater than those of the cryptorchid side. These differences were eliminated and, in some cases, even reversed in rams when the scrotal side was vasectomized. Differences between the ampullae in the calves were not as marked but favoured the scrotal side in each case. No differences were observed between the seminal vesicles or bulbo-urethrals from the two sides.

DISCUSSION

It is apparent from these experiments that in the ram and bull calf the androgen content of the unilateral cryptorchid testis is greatly reduced. In the ram the testosterone concentration in the two testes was similar, which supports the findings of Skinner et al. (1968) that in this species total hormone production depends upon the size of gonad. There was some indication that androstenedione might become the predominant androgen in retained ram testes which also supports the concept (Skinner et al. 1968) that the change in ratio between androstenedione and testosterone occurs during foetal life. In the calf, androstenedione remains the predominant androgen in the cryptorchid testis after 16 weeks of age, with a ratio of androstenedione:testosterone of $1:0.5$, in contrast to the contralateral scrotal testis in which the ratio was $1:5.5$. However, when a testis was returned to the abdomen at 8 months, after the time when testosterone has become the predominant androgen (Lindner & Mann, 1960), and left for 16 weeks, then testosterone remains the predominant androgen and although the concentration of both steroids was reduced in the cryptorchid testis the ratio remained similar. It is possible that the mature testis requires a longer intra-abdominal period before androstenedione becomes predominant. On the other hand, it is also possible that the mechanism whereby testosterone finally becomes dominant in the pubescent calf testis cannot be reversed by this treatment after a certain age.

There was some indication that in the unilaterally cryptorchid ram hormone production in the contralateral scrotal testis may have been improved. When the scrotal testes from the five rams unilaterally cryptorchidized were compared with bilateral scrotal testes from rams of similar age (from Skinner et al. 1968) in Table 2, it was noteworthy that they were larger and had a higher hormone concentration. The results must, however, be interpreted with caution as numbers were limited. There were breed differences and seasonal differences, although the latter were minimal for the two groups concerned. Nevertheless, this observation is in agreement with other reports on unilateral scrotal testes in pubescent animals (Ribbert, 1890; Lipschütz, 1922; Lindner & Rowson, 1961; Clegg, 1965 a, c).

The histochemistry of the interstitium, despite an apparent hypertrophy, indicated a markedly reduced activity in the cryptorchid testes. There was a lowered Δ^5-3β-hydroxysteroid dehydrogenase activity and very little lipid in the interstitium of the cryptorchid testis when compared with the control. These findings are in agreement with those of other workers (Llaurado & Dominguez, 1963; Kormano et al. 1964) and Hall (1965) found in vitro that steroid biosynthesis was significantly lower at $40°$ than at lower temperatures. In addition, the present study provides evidence in support of Moore's (1924b) suggestion that the apparent hypertrophy of the interstitium in cryptorchid testes was due to shrinkage of the seminiferous tubules.

Oslund (1926) first noted that supporting cells did not differentiate into Sertoli cells and this has been confirmed. Moreover, in contrast to findings in mature rats rendered cryptorchid (Lynch & Scott, 1951; Clegg, 1965b) there was very little lipid in the seminiferous tubules of pubescent cryptorchid testes.

When the testes were returned to the scrotum after 8 weeks and left for a further 8 weeks before autopsy, there was a degree of recovery. Not only had the hormone content increased as a result of increased testicular weight and the androstenedione: testosterone ratio widened, but there was some evidence of spermatogenesis. Further studies are required, for longer periods, before definite conclusions can be drawn, but it would appear that orchiopexy could lead to a large measure of testicular recovery provided the cryptorchid testis is normal and the operation is performed when the animals are young enough. As regards temperature effects on spermatogenesis, it is worth noting that in cultures grown at different temperatures, best maintenance of germinal cells and tubule structure was achieved at temperatures lower than $37°$ (Steinberger, Steinberger & Perloff, 1964). Seminiferous tubule diameter had doubled in both the scrotal and replaced testis, in contrast to testes cryptorchid for 16 weeks. This had already been shown to be a most useful parameter of sexual function in the ram (Skinner et al. 1968). The replaced testes were, in each case, surrounded by a large 'wad' of fat. There is little doubt that such testes were insulated by this fat and as insulation is known to affect spermatogenesis adversely (Moore & Oslund, 1924; Glover, 1956) recovery may have been more marked without the fat.

On the cryptorchid side the epididymis and vas deferens were greatly reduced in weight and size; the ampulla weighed less, was shorter and had a smaller diameter, and contained less fructose and citric acid. These differences were significant. The seminal vesicles and bulbo-urethral glands were unaffected.

In contrast to the findings of Tamura & Crew (1926), but in agreement with other authors (Moore & Quick, 1924b; Oslund, 1924; Cunningham, 1927) vasectomy had, by itself, no apparent effect on testicular histology or spermatogenesis, nor did it influence testicular hormone content. However, the latter observation was made on a pooled sample of testicular tissue and requires confirmation. On the vasectomized side the epididymis was distended with fluid with a consequent increase in size and weight, which agrees with the observation of Moore & Quick (1924b) in the rabbit. The ampulla on the vasectomized side was smaller than that on the other side whether cryptorchid or scrotal, and contained less fructose and citric acid. The seminal vesicles and bulbo-urethral glands were not affected by unilateral vasectomy.

From these experiments it appeared that even in the presence of the scrotal testis, the severance of the anatomical connexion between that testis and the vas deferens prevents the normal development of the ampulla. Presumably some testosterone must normally pass along the vas deferens in the testicular fluid and influence in this way the development of the ampulla.

We would like to thank Dr H. M. Dott and Professor T. Mann for reading the manuscript and for their interest in this work; Mr W. D. Booth and Dr R. V. Short

166

for assistance with the androgen determinations and Dr Mary Hay for advice on the histology. One of us (J.D.S.) is indebted for a scholarship to British Petroleum (Southern Africa).

REFERENCES

Antliff, H. R. & Young, W. C. (1957). Internal secretory capacity of the abdominal testis in the guinea pig. *Endocrinology* **61**, 121–127.

Bouin, P. & Ancel, P. (1903). Recherches sur les cellules interstitielles du testicule des mammifères. *Archs Zool. exp. gén.* **1**, 437–523.

Clegg, E. J. (1960). Some effects of artificial cryptorchidism on the accessory reproductive organs of the rat. *J. Endocr.* **20**, 210–219.

Clegg, E. J. (1961). Further studies on artificial cryptorchidism: quantitative changes in the interstitial cells of the rat testis. *J. Endocr.* **21**, 433–441.

Clegg, E. J. (1965*a*). Studies on artificial cryptorchidism: degenerative and regenerative changes in the germinal epithelium of the rat testis. *J. Endocr.* **33**, 259–268.

Clegg, E. J. (1965*b*). Studies on artificial cryptorchidism: histological appearances of unilateral and bilateral abdominal testes in the rat. *J. Endocr.* **33**, 269–278.

Clegg, E. J. (1965*c*). Compensatory changes in the scrotal testes of unilaterally cryptorchid rats. *J. Anat.* **99**, 417.

Crew, F. A. E. (1922). A suggestion as to the cause of the aspermatic condition of the imperfectly descended testis. *J. Anat.* **56**, 98–106.

Cunningham, J. T. (1927). Experiments on artificial cryptorchidism and ligature of the vas deferens in mammals. *Br. J. exp. Biol.* **4**, 333–341.

Engberg, H. (1949). Investigations on the endocrine function of the testicle in cryptorchidism. *Proc. R. Soc. Med.* **42**, 652–655.

Glover, T. D. (1956). The effect of scrotal insulation and the influence of breeding season upon fructose concentration in the semen of the ram. *J. Endocr* **13**, 235–242.

Griffiths, J. (1893). The structural changes in the testis of the dog when it is replaced within the abdominal cavity. *J. Anat. Physiol., Lond.* **27**, 482–499.

Hall, P. F. (1965). Influence of temperature upon the biosynthesis of testosterone by rabbit testis *in vitro*. *Endocrinology* **76**, 396–402.

Hanes, F. M. & Hooker, C. W. (1937). Hormone production in the undescended testis. *Proc. Soc. exp. Biol. Med.* **35**, 549–550.

Hay, M. F. & Deane, H. W. (1966). Attempts to demonstrate 3β- and 17β-hydroxysteroid dehydrogenase histochemically in the testes of the stallion, boar, ram and bull. *J. Reprod. Fert.* **12**, 551–560.

Jeffries, M. E. (1931). Hormone production by experimental cryptorchid rat testes as indicated by the seminal vesicle and prostate cytology tests. *Anat. Rec.* **48**, 131–137.

Kimeldorf, D. J. (1948). Excretion of 17-ketosteroids by male rabbits during altered gonadal function. *Endocrinology* **43**, 83–88.

Kormano, M., Harkonen, M. & Kontinen, E. (1964). Effect of experimental cryptorchidism on the histochemically demonstrable dehydrogenases of the rat testis. *Endocrinology* **74**, 44–51.

Lindner, H. R. & Mann, T. (1960). Relationship between the content of androgenic steroids in the testes and the secretory activity of the seminal vesicles in the bull. *J. Endocr.* **21**, 341–360.

Lindner, H. R. & Rowson, L. E. A. (1961). Androgens and related compounds in the spermatic vein blood of domestic animals. III. The effect of unilateral orchidectomy on the rate of androgen secretion by the remaining testis in the immature calf. *J. Endocr.* **23**, 167–170.

Lipschütz, A. (1922). The so-called compensatory hypertrophy of the testicle after unilateral castration. *J. Physiol., Lond.* **66**, 451–458.

Llaurado, J. G. & Dominguez, O. V. (1963). Effect of cryptorchidism on testicular enzymes involved in androgen biosynthesis. *Endocrinology* **72**, 292–295.

Lynch, K. M. & Scott, W. W. (1951). Lipid distribution in the Sertoli cell and Leydig cell of the rat testis as related to experimental alterations in the pituitary-gonad system. *Endocrinology* **49**, 8–14.

Mann, T., Rowson, L. E. A., Short, R. V. & Skinner, J. D. (1967). The relationship between nutrition and androgenic activity in pubescent twin calves, and the effect of orchitis. *J. Endocr.* **38**, 455–468.

Moore, C. R. (1924*a*). The behaviour of the testis in transplantation, experimental cryptorchidism, vasectomy, scrotal insulation and heat application. *Endocrinology* **8**, 493–508.

Moore, C. R. (1924*b*). Testicular reactions in experimental cryptorchidism. *Am. J. Anat.* **34**, 269–316.

Moore, C. R. (1926). Scrotal replacement of experimental cryptorchid testes and the recovery of spermatogenic function. *Biol. Bull. mar. biol. Lab., Woods Hole* **51**, 112–128.

Moore, C. R. (1944). Hormone secretion by experimental cryptorchid testes. *Yale J. Biol. Med.* **17**, 203–216.

Moore, C. R. & Gallagher, T. F. (1930). Seminal vesicle and prostate function as a testis hormone indicator of the electric ejaculation test. *Am. J. Anat.* **45**, 39–70.

Moore, C. R. & Oslund, R. (1924). Experiments on the sheep testis: cryptorchidism, vasectomy and scrotal insulation. *Am. J. Physiol.* **67**, 595–607.

Moore, C. R. & Quick, W. J. (1924*a*). The scrotum as a temperature regulator for the testes. *Am. J. Physiol.* **68**, 70–79.

Moore, C. R. & Quick, W. J. (1924*b*). Vasectomy in the rabbit. *Am. J. Anat.* **34**, 317–336.

Morehead, J. R. & Morgan, C. F. (1967). Hormone production by experimental cryptorchid rat testes as indicated by radioautographic studies of the seminal vesicles and coagulating glands. *Fert. Steril.* **18**, 232–237.

Nelson, W. O. (1937). Some factors involved in the control of the gametogenic and endocrine function of the testis. *Cold Spring Harb. Symp. quant. Biol.* **5**, 123–135.

Oslund, R. (1924). A study of vasectomy on rats and guinea pigs. *Am. J. Physiol.* **67**, 422–443.

Oslund, R. M. (1926). Cryptorchid testes and testicular hormone production. *Am. J. Physiol.* **77**, 76–82.

Ribbert, — (1890). Ueber die compensatorische Hypertrophie der Geschlechtsdrüsen. *Virchows Arch. path. Anat. Physiol.* **120**, 247–272.

Sand, K. (1921). Etudes expérimentales sur les glandes sexuelles chez les mammifères cryptorchidie expérimentale. *J. Physiol. Path. gén.* **19**, 515–527.

Skinner, J. D., Booth, W. D., Rowson, L. E. A. & Karg, H. (1968). The postnatal development of the reproductive tract of the Suffolk ram, and changes in the gonadotrophin content of the pituitary. *J. Reprod. Fert.* (In the Press.)

Skinner, J. D. & Rowson, L. E. A. (1967). Effect of unilateral cryptorchidism on sexual development in the pubescent male animal. *J. Reprod. Fert.* **14**, 349–350.

Steinberger, A. A., Steinberger, E. & Perloff, W. H. (1964). Mammalian testes in organ culture. *Expl Cell Res.* **36**, 19–27.

Tamura, Y. & Crew, F. A. E. (1926). On effects of vasectomy and of epididymodefentectomy in the mouse. *Proc. R. Soc. Edinb.* **46**, 285–288.

Threadgold, L. T. (1957). Sudan black and osmic acid as staining agents for testicular interstitial cells. *Stain Technol.* **32**, 267–270.

DESCRIPTION OF PLATES

PLATE 1

The reproductive tracts of two lambs, 16 weeks after the left testis had been made unilaterally cryptorchid. One of the lambs (on the left) was also vasectomized at the same time as it was made cryptorchid. Note that after vasectomy there was no apparent difference in size between the ampullae. Note also the smaller ampulla on the cryptorchid side compared with the contralateral 'scrotal' ampulla in the tract on the right. Abbreviations: A = ampulla; B = bulbo-urethral glands; CE = cauda epididymis; SV = seminal vesicles; T = testis; VD = vas deferens.

PLATE 2

Figs. 1, 2. Unfixed frozen sections from the testes of an experimental, unilaterally cryptorchid calf incubated for 3 hr. to demonstrate Δ^5-3β-hydroxysteroid dehydrogenase activity. There was less activity in the cryptorchid testis (fig. 1) after 16 weeks than in the contralateral scrotal testis (fig. 2). ($\times$110.)

Figs. 3, 4. Paraffin sections from the testes of the same calf showing interstitial cells. There was very little lipid in the interstitium of the cryptorchid testis (fig. 3) when compared to the contralateral scrotal testis (fig. 4). Sudan black. ($\times$110.)

Figs. 5, 6. Unfixed frozen sections from the testes of a 3-yr.-old natural unilateral cryptorchid stallion showing NADPH diaphorase activity. This activity was mainly within the tubules of the cryptorchid testis (fig. 5) and in the interstitium of the contralateral scrotal testis (fig. 6). Incubation time 1 hr. ($\times$110.)

Figs. 7, 8. Unfixed frozen sections from the testes of a calf made unilaterally cryptorchid incubated for 1 hr. to demonstrate NADPH diaphorase activity. The left testis had been cryptorchid for 16 weeks (fig. 7) and diaphorase activity was still mainly in the interstitium, as in the contralateral scrotal testis (fig. 8). ($\times$110.)

Transverse sections stained with Delafield's haematoxylin and chromotrope 2 R.

Figs. 9, 10. Testes of a 2-yr.-old natural unilateral cryptorchid ram. Note the single layer of supporting cells and no gonocytes in the seminiferous tubules of the cryptorchid testis (fig. 9). The contralateral scrotal testis (fig. 10) shows all stages of spermatogenesis. ($\times$400.)

168

Plate 1

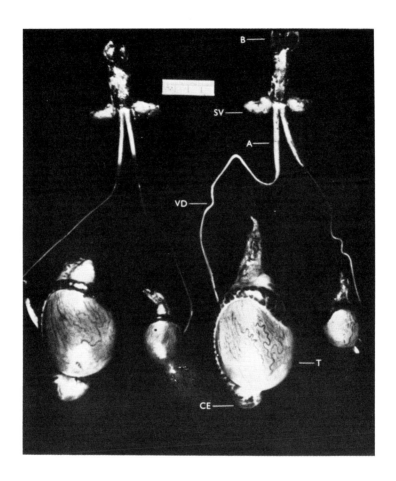

Plate 2

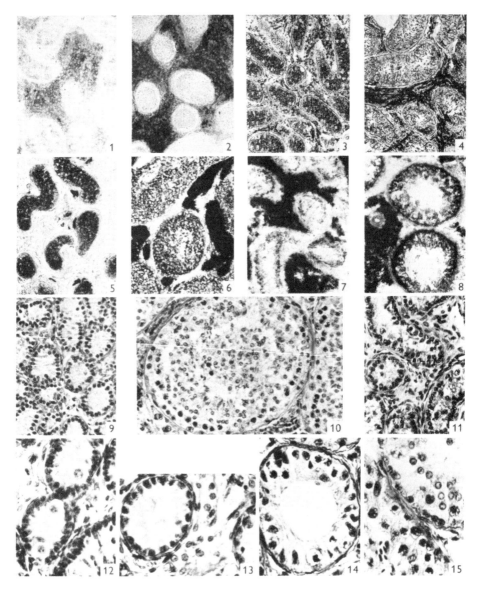

Fig. 11. Testis of a 16-week-old lamb made unilaterally cryptorchid. Note the single layer of supporting cells and the presence of gonocytes in the seminiferous tubules of the cryptorchid testis. Spermatogenesis was normal in the contralateral scrotal testis. (× 400.)

Figs. 12, 13. After 8 weeks in the abdomen, supporting cells and gonocytes were still present in the seminiferous tubules of the cryptorchid testis (fig. 12), but tubule diameter was much smaller than in the contralateral scrotal testis (fig. 13). (× 640.)

Figs. 14, 15. Eight weeks after return to the scrotum, spermatogenesis had started in the formerly cryptorchid testis (fig. 14), the tubules had doubled in size and a lumen had formed. In the contralateral scrotal testis (fig. 15), spermatogenesis was further advanced, spermatids were abundant and some were in the final stages of spermiogenesis; the diameter of the tubules was also larger. (× 640.)

Reversal of Vasectomy

VASECTOMY FOR VOLUNTARY MALE STERILISATION

HOWARD G. HANLEY

M.D. Lpool, F.R.C.S.

RECENT HISTORY

BEFORE 1960 it was widely believed by British doctors that it was illegal to perform male sterilisation for reasons other than to protect a man's physical or mental health. In fact it has never been illegal,[1] though the operation was discouraged by the medical defence societies. In 1961 the annual report of the Medical Defence Union (on p. 13) indicated a change of attitude, and by 1965 the annual report (on p. 10) contained a modified form of consent to voluntary male sterilisation. Many hundreds of vasectomy operations have been performed since then, and provided that the safeguards suggested by the defence societies are adhered to most surgeons consider that acceptance has become a *fait accompli*.

Before 1965 most of the reports on voluntary male sterilisation came from abroad, and it was not until 1966 that the subject was discussed openly in the British journals, largely due to the influence of Blacker and Jackson.[2] At that time there were reports of several large series of vasectomy operations, but, though they devoted much space to the psychological and sociological advantages of the operation, conclusions about the clinical end-results were, with a few notable exceptions,[3][4] scanty, contradictory, or even non-existent. A few of these papers (e.g., that by Phadke[5]) contain a passing reference to some of the clinical problems which British surgeons are encountering today, but they were published in journals which the average British surgeon does not regularly read and might even have difficulty in obtaining.

Up to the present time I have been unable to find any good acceptable summary of world surgical opinion about the technique, morbidity, or long-term results of vasectomy, so that my present views are based upon my own experience. However, I have learnt much in two years, and most of it is contrary to accepted teaching.

1. Addison, P. H. *Br. med. J.* 1968, ii, 702
2. Blacker, C. P., Jackson, L. N. *Lancet*, 1966, i, 971.
3. O'Connor, V. J. *J. Am. med. Ass.* 1948, 136, 162.
4. Rolnick, H. C. *J. Urol.* 1934, 72, 915.
5. Phadke, G. M. *J. Indian med. Ass.* 1961, 37, 241.

In most instances it is wise to restrict the performance of vasectomy to couples who are judged to be stable, and happily married, and who already have a family. I always insist on seeing both husband and wife together, so that I can assess the couple and can also obtain their written consent, signed and witnessed in each other's presence. It is important to explain to both of them that the male is not sterile for about three months after the operation, during which period contraceptives must continue to be used, and even then not until at least two semen counts have been shown to be azoospermic. (After the operation it is most important to again remind the couple of these points. Incidentally, since we are not interested in sperm motility, a condom specimen remains perfectly satisfactory for counting purposes for about 48 hours, so that a specimen sent through the post is perfectly adequate.) It should also be emphasised that the operation will not affect potency or libido. I personally perform the operation in such a way that reanastomosis can be attempted if required, and I always tell the patient this fact, adding that nevertheless there is only about a 50% chance of success.

SURGICAL TECHNIQUE

The possibility that a divided vas could rejoin spontaneously was suggested by several workers, especially O'Connor[3] and Rolnick,[4] but most surgeons rather doubted these observations. Only a few years ago any British general surgeon assumed that he knew how to tie the vas—he had done it hundreds of times during prostatic surgery—and, though each surgeon uses a different technique, no-one would admit that he did it inefficiently. The fact that a vas could recanalise after it had been divided and ligatured would still be doubted by some surgeons today. If a piece was actually removed, spontaneous rejoining might be considered even more impossible. However, we now know that spontaneous rejoining can occur unless very special precautions are used to prevent it.[6] There are undoubtedly many ways of preventing this rejoining and it is obvious that the ideal operation has not yet been devised—but it was ever thus in surgery.

It seems that simple division and ligature, or even the resection of two to three centimetres of the vas, will not prevent recanalisation if the divided ends are allowed to come into alignment again, and this we[6] have proved by microscopic examination of the tissue removed at a second operation. In practice, it is very difficult to destroy the mucosa and to seal the ends of the divided vas. Simple

6. Hanley, H. G., Pugh, R. C. B. *Br. J. Urol.* (in the press).

175

crushing still leaves areas of epithelial cells, and these can produce a fistula anywhere in the body. Occlusion with catgut can only be temporary, while silk or nylon cut through easily. Diathermy fulguration, though probably effective in destroying the mucosa temporarily, can cause pain radiating into the iliac fossa for several days. This reaction is difficult to explain, but can be very troublesome to the patient.

Since one can never be sure of occluding the severed ends of the vas by simple mechanical means, I think that the only way of preventing recanalisation is to keep them well apart. In practice it is difficult to prevent the ends being drawn into contact again in much the same way as the ends of a long bone are drawn into contact by contraction of the surrounding soft structures, and, because the dartos muscles are very well developed in some men, the cords may shorten strikingly for a time immediately after operation. One such example (fig. 1, left) shows how the two ends were drawn together again, despite removal of a 1 cm. length of vas. A series of sections through the nodule, studied by my colleague Dr. R. C. B. Pugh, showed epithelial areas inside the scar tissue, and the patient continued to have spermatozoa in the ejaculate for eleven months, until this segment of vas was removed and the ends turned back. It is obvious that if sufficient vas is removed the ends cannot come into contact again, and Wallace [6] recommends the removal of several inches. However, I am concerned not only with achieving a complete azoospermia but in being able to rejoin the vas at a later

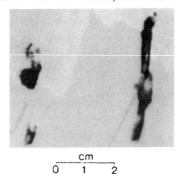

cm
0   1   2

Right   Left

Fig. 1—A pair of vasa, excised following previous vasectomy, showing nodules of scar tissue.

date if necessary, and therefore I try to preserve as much of the vas as possible. The most practical way of avoiding recanalisation is to prevent the ends of the vas coming into contact again: to do this the ends must be separated by physical barriers, such as tissue planes, or by deliberately ensuring that the open ends point away from each other. Rolnick [4] achieved this by folding the ends of the vas back upon themselves, while lately I have on occasion been overlapping the two ends so that the openings point in opposite directions (fig. 2). I use fine chromic catgut and avoid tying this too tightly, so that it does not cut into the lumen of the vas.

176

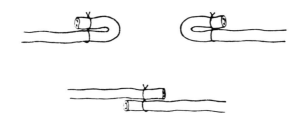

Fig. 2—Two methods of ensuring that the divided ends of the vasa do not come into contact or alignment.

Reanastomosis after such a procedure is a fairly simple operation with a high success-rate, and the time-interval between vasectomy and reanastomosis does not in my experience affect the chances of success. The longest interval was nine years, and sperms appeared in the ejaculate three weeks after the reanastomosis.

SOME PERSONAL OBSERVATIONS

Many thousands of male sterilisations have been performed,[7] but detailed long-term follow-up records are difficult to obtain, so that a small series with adequate data may be of value.

Double Vasa

I have seen nearly 100 cases of absence of the vas in twenty years, but double vasa must be very rare indeed, and I have not seen a case over the same period. None of my close urological colleagues has encountered a case, and the anatomy has never been reported in detail.

Sperm Storage

Surgeons interested in male fertility have always been concerned with the site of sperm storage. We have been told in the past that sperms are not normally stored in the vesicles, but are retained in the epididymis until the erectile phase, when they are passed down the vas to the ampulla. This is supported by findings in patients with bilateral tuberculosis of the seminal vesicles, in whom the total sperm numbers may remain unaltered despite a slowly decreasing volume of ejaculate fluid. I have seen this diminution of volume progress to the stage when there was insufficient fluid to carry sperms to the meatus, but when millions of sperms could be obtained by gentle rectal urethral massage after orgasm.

Nevertheless I now have to revise my opinions in the light of experience following vasectomy. There is no doubt whatever that regardless of where the sperms are stored below the point of occlusion they remain living in

---

7. Family Planning News, August to November, 1965, p. 24. Ministry of Health, New Delhi.

large numbers and will appear in the semen after many ejaculations over many months. In 1 man sperms were still present after thirty-two ejaculations.

In a small carefully controlled series of 7 patients—all professional men—a condom specimen of every ejaculate was examined until azoospermia was achieved. In every case, second or third specimens showed a striking drop in density, but there was a more gradual drop from then onwards. In this particular group, the earliest azoospermia occurred after six ejaculations, and the latest after twelve; there is obviously a very great individual variation.

In another consecutive series of 75 patients the shortest recorded interval before azoospermia was three weeks (eight ejaculations), and the longest was seventeen weeks (about ten ejaculations). Not every ejaculate specimen was examined in this series, but it seems that the number of ejaculations is more important than the time-interval in achieving azoospermia, and this should be explained to the patient. 1 of my patients abstained for six weeks and then recorded a count of about 40 million per ml. Fortunately he rapidly became azoospermic when the situation was explained to him.

The presence of large numbers of sperms six to eight weeks after operation is suspicious of recanalisation, because in most of my patients sperms were reduced to a few per high-power field after five or six ejaculations (three weeks), and only an occasional sperm was seen at two months. An occasional sperm after four to five months is highly suspicious, but not conclusive of failure. This makes it very difficult to pronounce upon complete azoospermia—rationally only 1 sperm is necessary, and you may not see it. Most of these examinations were made on condom specimens, so that I do not have any reliable evidence about sperm motility as opposed to numbers, but many live sperms were present in one fresh specimen seven weeks after operation and in another after twelve ejaculations in ten weeks. The patient must be completely azoospermic before he can be considered sterile.

Recanalisation of the Divided Vas

Although I realised that the vas could rejoin if the open ends were in contact, until lately I firmly believed that they must be rejoined very shortly after operation, before the two ends became sealed off, and assumed that when the postoperative sperm-count finally became negative the patient was permanently sterile. However, if the two severed ends are in alignment anything can happen. A patient who had one azoospermic test many weeks after vasectomy made his wife pregnant about ten months after the azoospermic specimen, at which time two positive counts were recorded.[8] Rolnick[4] thought that regeneration was possible after many years. This regenerative process has now been confirmed microscopically by Dr. Pugh, who has lately shown that crushing or tight ligaturing may liberate epithelial cells which can proliferate as islands of mucosa, and that these can in turn join together to eventually form an epithelial-lined channel.[6] The distance over which this can occur, and the time-interval required, is unknown, but it can only be repeated that at vasectomy every effort must be made to separate the ends of the vas by tissue planes or to point them in opposite directions.

Morbidity

Many reported operations have been performed under local anæsthetic, most probably done as day cases. However, I have abandoned local in favour of a general anæsthetic and am now most reluctant to allow patients home the same day. There is no doubt that if all goes well the operation can be rendered painless by local anæsthetic, but if the cord is thick and the vas difficult to isolate, or if bleeding (which cannot possibly be predicted or prevented) is troublesome, an embarrassing situation can arise. It is true that in scrotal surgery a hæmatoma usually develops within a few hours or not at all, but this is not an infallible rule, and in my experience the best protection against a hæmatoma is to ensure that the patient remains *asleep* for several hours so that he cannot examine the operation-site. This can be achieved by a general anæsthetic with adequate preoperative and postoperative sedation. If the patient is allowed home the same day there is a very definite risk of a secondary hæmatoma; in 3 personal cases the scrotum was normal when the patient was discharged 7 or 8 hours after operation, but a hæmatoma developed during the journey home (1 by train, 2 by motor-car). Stidolph[9] has 2 patients who developed hæmatomata five and seven days after operation. This operation, though simple in theory, can be embarrassing in practice, and is not without morbidity, which can be reduced by the regimen I have described.

If a large hæmatoma should develop I would evacuate it as soon as possible by opening up the scrotum. Aspiration is useless, while " leaving well alone " may leave the patient with a painful swollen mass for many weeks.

Reanastomosis

My own series of 32 patients includes a group of 13 men who were sterilised in prison camps. 3 operations had

---

8. Wallace, D. M. Personal communication.
9. Stidolph, N. Personal communication.

179

been performed without an anæsthetic of any kind; in one case both epididymal tails had been completely destroyed, probably by crushing, while in another, in which inguinal incisions had been used, the upper ends of the vasa could not be found. In another man so much vas had been removed that the anastomosis was under too much tension to have any hope of success. Despite these problems sperms appeared in the ejaculate after reanastomosis in 8 of the 13 men (61%), the earliest positive count being within three weeks of operation, though sperms may have been present before this. The youngest patient in this group at the time of vasectomy was thirteen, the oldest twenty-nine years. The time-interval between vasectomy and reanastomosis varied between one year and nine years. My average success-rate for the appearance of spermatozoa after a technically satisfactory anastomosis is well over 70%. The word " success " requires qualification in that sperms in the ejaculate do not necessarily mean a pregnancy. One of the most important factors is the age of the patient, and more especially that of his wife, at the time of reanastomosis.

In my later series of 19 men, in whom reanastomosis was performed after deliberate voluntary vasectomy, or accidental surgical injury (3 bilateral hernias, 2 bilateral hydrocele operations), the average age of the patients was over forty. I have also operated on 4 patients with bilateral hernia injuries in whom the upper ends of the vasa could not be found at the internal ring, so that anastomotic surgery was impossible. 2 of these patients had originally been operated on before the age of five, and 1 at about twelve years. The 4th man had undergone an apparently deliberate closure of the inguinal canals for bilateral recurrent herniæ; though no trace of a vascular cord or vas could be found near the site of the internal inguinal ring in this patient, both testes were viable, and living spermatozoa were present in the epididymal heads. The collateral circulation at this level is obviously excellent. (In the patient who had originally been operated upon at the age of twelve an attempt was made to find the vas within the abdomen; this procedure is not recommended.) To place these 9 accidental surgical injuries in proper perspective it should be mentioned that, though I have not examined my subfertility records in detail, many dozens of inguinal scars have been explored in the hope of finding a reparable traumatic injury of the vas, but only in these 9 men was a previous operation responsible for the azoospermia. Unilateral injury may be common, but bilateral injury is not.

Age in itself reduces the chances of a pregnancy, even when sperms are present in the ejaculate. Most of the men seeking reanastomosis after voluntary ligation had a grown-up family by a previous marriage; such men of

40–50 fall into a notoriously subfertile group well recognised by clinicians interested in male subfertility.

CONCLUSIONS

Vasectomy is an excellent form of male sterilisation, but it is not a light-hearted minor operation. It carries a failure and a morbidity rate, but with reasonable care and attention to detail these can be reduced to acceptable levels. It cannot be stressed too often that the man is not sterile for several months after the operation, and that even then his azoospermia must be confirmed microscopically.

SPONTANEOUS RECANALISATION OF THE DIVIDED VAS DEFERENS

By R. C. B. PUGH, M.D., F.C.Path., and HOWARD G. HANLEY, M.D., F.R.C.S.

VOLUNTARY male sterilisation with the object of producing complete sterility without loss of potency or libido is best achieved by carefully performed bilateral vasectomy. The operation is not technically difficult, but it is perhaps not sufficiently widely appreciated that spontaneous recanalisation of the divided vasa sometimes occurs subsequently, with the return of the sperm count to normal or near normal values (O'Connor, 1948; Rolnick, 1954; Bunge, 1968).

This paper reports a series of seven patients in whom the vasa recanalised after complete surgical section, in some cases combined with partial excision.

Case Histories.—Seven healthy adult males had been subjected to bilateral vasectomy in order to render them sterile. In three men (Group I) a segment of vas, up to 3 or 4 cm. in length, had been excised and the cut ends tied off, and in the other four (Group II) the vasa had merely been divided and tied. Routine post-operative examinations of ejaculates were carried out. The operation was deemed to have failed in all seven either when a patient's wife became pregnant or because sperms continued to be found in the ejaculate for longer than the three to five month period usually considered necessary to empty the vesicles (Hanley, 1968). The findings are summarised in the Table.

All seven patients were re-explored (Case 1 by Mr P. Hickinbotham of Leicester General Hospital, and the remainder by H. G. H.) and segments of vas were removed from each side.

Pathology.—The specimens available for pathological examination consisted of paraffin-embedded material of the portions of the right and left vasa excised at the first operation in Case 1, and the lengths of vas removed at the second operation in each of the seven patients. The pieces of vas were pinned out on to sheet cork immediately after removal, care being taken to avoid placing pins through narrow segments or nodular areas. The cork was then floated, with the specimen on its underside, on the surface of a bowl of formol saline to ensure fixation without undue distortion. After adequate fixation the specimens were photographed and any narrowed or dilated or otherwise obviously abnormal areas were embedded in paraffin and sectioned serially (Cases 1, 4, 5 and 7), or by the step-section technique (Cases 2, 3 and 6).

RESULTS

Group I (vasectomy with resection)

Case 1.—The portions of the right and left vasa excised at the first operation were of normal appearance (Fig. 1). The specimens received from the second operation are illustrated in Figure 2. The piece of right vas measured 9·5 cm. in length and had a uniform external diameter of 0·25 cm. except in the centre, where there was an irregular expanded area 1 cm. in length and up to 0·6 cm. in diameter. The piece of left vas was 8·5 cm. long and was similarly thickened in one area. Serial 5 μ sections in the transverse plane were examined from the scarred areas of the vasa and several random transverse sections were taken above and below the scars. These latter sections revealed an essentially normal appearance, similar to that seen in Figure 1. The findings in the scarred areas are shown in diagrammatic form in Figure 3. The first operation had clearly been successful on the left side because many of the cross-sections passed through fibrous tissue only, or through fibrous tissue and muscle (Fig. 4). Vas epithelium was found in a few, but by no means all, of the cross-sections and continuity had clearly not been re-established on this side. In contrast vas epithelium was found at all levels in the scar tissue on the right side. Sections near to the limits of the macroscopically obvious scar showed considerable thickening due to a mass of well-vascularised collagen surrounding an apparently normal vas. As the level of surgical section was

Summary of Clinical Findings

Primary Procedure	Case No.	Follow-up	Time interval between Primary Procedure and Re-exploration
Group I Vasa resected and tied	1	6 million sperms in ejaculate at 6 weeks, and 86 million at 13 weeks post-operatively.	10 months
	2	Sperms in ejaculate at 4 and 12 months post-operatively.	16 months
	3	Azoospermic at 2 months after operation. Wife pregnant 10 months after vasectomy. Sperms in ejaculate when wife found to be pregnant.	18 months
Group II Vasa cut and tied	4	Occasional sperms at 3 months and many at 4 months post-vasectomy.	5 months
	5	Sperms in ejaculate at 5 months.	6 months
	6	Azoospermic at 10 and 12 weeks after vasectomy. Wife pregnant at 10 months; sperms in ejaculate when wife found to be pregnant.	9 months
	7	Wife pregnant within one month of vasectomy. An occasional sperm present at the second operation.	3 months

approached the vas, while still maintaining the normal relations of its epithelium and muscle, showed marked budding of the epithelium (Fig. 5), the buds and tubules penetrating the muscle coats and reaching the collagenous tissue surrounding the muscle and binding the two cut ends of the vas together (Fig. 6). As the sections were traced towards the centre of the scar, vas epithelium was seen in every cross-section either as a small apparently solid bud of cells or, much more commonly, as a small tubule. Muscle bundles, as illustrated in Figure 4, also occurred and were sometimes, but by no means invariably, adjacent to the epithelial elements. They were most numerous in the sections taken through the peripheral parts of the scarred areas. Occasionally old small sperm granulomas were seen in the depths of the scar, often close to the segments of vas epithelium. The deltaic proliferation of vas epithelium was seen immediately proximally and distally to the scarred area, as indicated in Figure 3, and had given rise to the vasal elements which were seen in the denser central parts of the scar. This was considered to indicate that reconstitution of the vas had occurred.

Case 2.—The two pieces of vas each measured 3 cm. in length and were between 0·3 and 0·4 cm. in external diameter with areas of thickening up to 0·8 cm. in diameter in their central parts. It was found on sectioning that no lumen or vas epithelium was seen in the dense scar tissue on the right side and it was assumed, therefore, that the first operation had been successful on this side. However, in every section examined on the left side, patent vas or small tubules of vas epithelium or sperm granulomata were seen. These findings, together with the fact that the ejaculate contained sperms, were considered sufficient to indicate that continuity had been re-established on this side.

Case 3.—The resected portion of right vas measured 4·2 cm. in length and step-sectioning revealed complete interruption of the vas by dense scar tissue, with some residual suture material in the outer areas of the scar in

183

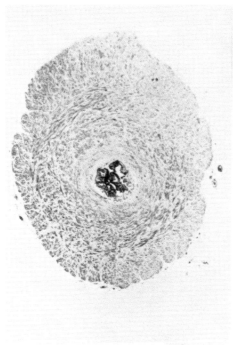

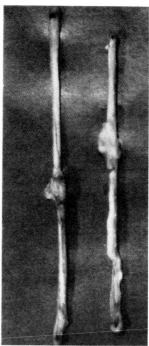

FIG. 1   FIG. 2

—— Muscle of Vas

⫶⫶⫶ Epithelium of Vas

⫶⫶⫶ Scar

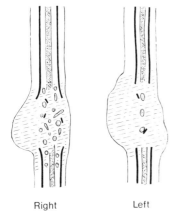

Right   Left

FIG. 3

Fig. 1.—Case 1.—Cross-section of the piece of normal right vas excised at the first operation. Note the well-developed muscle coats arranged in three layers. (H. & E. × 40.)

Fig. 2.—Case 1.—Portions of vasa excised at the second operation. (×1·2).

Fig. 3.—Case 1.—Diagram of the findings on serial sectioning of the scarred areas seen in Figure 2.

184

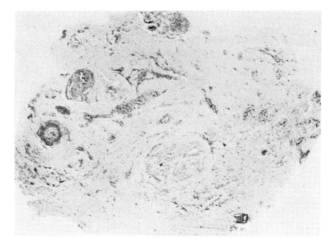

FIG. 4

Case 1.—Cross-section of scar in left vas (second operation). Some muscle bundles can be seen just below right centre but the bulk of the section consists of well vascularised fibrous tissue. No vas epithelium can be identified. (H & E. ×40.)

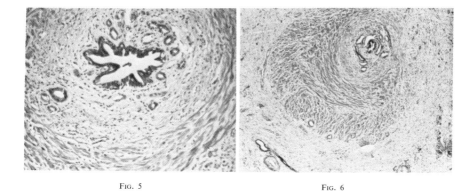

FIG. 5   FIG. 6

Fig. 5.—Case 1.—Right vas. The epithelium has proliferated, with the formation of many small tubules in the lamina propria. (H & E. ×128.)

Fig. 6.—Case 1.—Right vas. There is marked proliferation of vas epithelium in the lamina propria and small tubules are also seen in the outer muscle and adventitia. (H. & E. ×48.)

several areas. The piece of left vas was 2·6 cm. in length with an area of nodular thickening centrally. Step-sections revealed epithelial-lined channels at all levels examined with sperm heads within them and also within the surrounding scar tissue. Sperms were found in the lumen of the vas at each end of the specimen that was excised, thus clearly demonstrating that recanalisation must have occurred.

Group II (vasa cut and tied off)

Case 4.—Each piece of vas measured 0·7 cm. in length and 0·4 cm. in external diameter with a terminal expansion into a firm light yellow coloured nodule 0·5 cm. in diameter. Microscopically one of these yellow nodules was shown by serial sections to be a sperm granuloma in which there was a complex mass of proliferating fibroblastic and fibrous tissues with many small tubules lined by vasal epithelium and irregular clefts and spaces lined by a simple or pseudo-stratified epithelium. In the other specimen the nodule contained no structures which could be identified as having been derived from the vas epithelium, and it consisted only of well-vascularised fibromuscular tissue focally infiltrated with chronic inflammatory cells and containing pigment macrophages. Recanalisation was therefore thought to have occurred through the first of the step terminal nodules, but not the other.

Case 5.—The fragments of right and left vas measured respectively 2·5 and 1·2 cm. in length and were constricted centrally (Fig. 7). Serial sectioning of the narrowed areas showed a central epithelial lined channel with sperm heads in the lumen in all sections on the left side but complete interruption of the vas by scar tissue on the right.

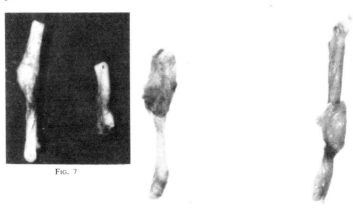

FIG. 7

FIG. 8

Fig. 7.—Case 5.—Resected portions of vasa each showing well marked central constriction and scarring. (×1·9).

Fig. 8.—Case 6.—Resected pieces of vasa showing the localised areas of thickening and scarring. (×1·5).

Case 6.—The two pieces of vas measured 3·3 and 4·3 cm. in length and in each there was a thickened area (Fig. 8) at the site of the previous operation. On the right side there was complete disappearance of all vasal epithelium and muscle in the centre of the thickened zone, indicating that the transection had been complete and successful. On the left many vas epithelial elements were seen in all the step sections examined and there was a marked proliferation of the epithelium forming small acini and islets within the scar tissue similar to those seen in the right vas in Case 1 (see Figs. 3 and 6). It was concluded that recanalisation had occurred on the left side.

Case 7.—The piece of left vas measured 1·3 cm. in length and its external diameter varied between 0·3 cm. and 0·6 cm. The narrower end had the structure of normal vas but the broader end consisted of a mass of dense collagenous fibrous tissue focally infiltrated with chronic inflammatory cells, and as this contained no epithelial elements surgical section was thought to have been complete on this side. The portion of right vas was 1 × 1·5 × 0·5 cm. in its maximum dimensions and serial sectioning showed that part had a relatively normal outline and overall structure, though there were several sperm granulomata in the outer layers of its wall. In its broadest part the tissue contours were lost and a large sperm granuloma replaced the normal structure with muscle bundles, proliferated vas epithelium and masses of endothelioid cells surrounding dense clumps of sperm heads (Fig. 9). It was concluded that recanalisation had occurred on this side.

In summary, the histological examinations showed that recanalisation of one vas had occurred in each of the seven patients—three on the right side and three on the left; in one patient (Case 4) it was not known which vas had recanalised. There are distinct differences in the appearances

186

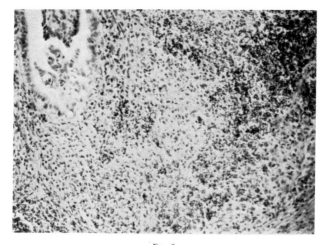

FIG. 9

Case 7.—Sperm granuloma at the plane of surgical section of the vas.
(H & E. × 160.)

between the Group I and the Group II cases, perhaps the most striking being the larger amount and greater density of the scar tissue in the Group I specimens. Also the sperm granulomas seen in the Group I cases were small and virtually effete, and consisted of collections of chronic inflammatory cells and a few macrophages with, occasionally, nuclear dust, whereas those in the Group II lesions were much larger and more florid, with many sperms—sometimes in vast numbers—and conglomerations of proliferated vas epithelial cells and macrophages, together with some fibroblastic tissue and muscle. The permeation of the scar tissue by anastomosing and branching tubules lined by vasal epithelium was a particular feature of the Group I cases.

DISCUSSION

The findings in this small series clearly show that what most surgeons regard as a simple operation—and one that is often classed as a minor procedure to be carried out on an outpatient under local anæsthesia—can sometimes have unforeseen results.

Recanalisation of the vas after vasectomy might be expected to occur if, at the conclusion of the operation, the epithelial cells of the two cut ends are allowed to come into contact. Experience shows that it is extremely difficult in practice to prevent this contact, and that adequate closure of the two ends may not be possible using any of the generally accepted surgical techniques (Hanley, 1968). Simple ligation, for example, is often ineffective because the vas is a thick-walled, muscular, semi-rigid tube which usually does not collapse completely when ligated. Furthermore, a catgut ligature will produce only temporary occlusion and a non-absorbable ligature, if tight enough to obliterate the lumen, may cut through. Diathermy destruction of the ends of the vas will produce scar tissue into which the cells of the vas epithelium may be displaced, and simple crushing may produce a similar state of affairs.

It has not been possible to demonstrate the full sequence of events leading to recanalisation of the vas in the present series of cases but it is likely that a situation develops not unlike that

187

which occurs after the fracture of a long bone. If there is any leakage of seminal fluid or local accumulation of tissue fluid, one or other, or both, cut ends of the vas will become surrounded by a sperm granuloma, in much the same way as a callus is formed around the ends of a fractured bone. There is evidence that this, in fact, occurred in all the Group II cases reported here. In these cases, too, a conspicuous feature was a very marked proliferation of the vas epithelium, forming sheets of cells which grew out into the granulomata. In this respect the lesions differ significantly from the not uncommon sperm granulomata seen in the region of the epididymis (Glassy and Mostofi, 1956; Phillips, 1961).

The appearances in the Group I cases, in which the time interval between the two operations was very much longer than in the Group II patients, are consistent with the granulomata having healed and formed scar tissue. There is nothing to suggest that the differences might in any way

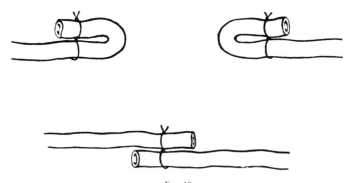

Fig. 10

Two methods of preventing the cut ends of the vas coming into contact after vasectomy.

be due to variations in the operative technique used in the initial operations. It is likely that the organisation and scarring of the granulomata occurred in much the same way as tuberculous lesions heal by fibrosis, but the stimulus which promoted the persistence and proliferation, and also the subsequent recanalisation, of the remnants of the vas epithelium is not known. The distance through which the epithelial cells can migrate is obviously limited, and excision of long pieces of vas (as in Case 1, Fig. 2) would clearly achieve the desired result and ensure permanent sterility. Removal of short pieces of vas is much less satisfactory because contraction of the cremasteric muscle fibres will tend to draw the cut ends together again and thus negate the effect of the excision. However, it is not unknown for a sterilised patient to ask that fertility be restored and it is therefore essential to compromise and to plan the sterilising procedure in such a way as not to jeopardise a re-anastomosing operation at a later date.

For this reason resection of long pieces of vas is to be avoided and much the best results are obtained either by placing the two cut ends in different fascial planes (which, incidentally, may be extremely difficult) or by folding the cut ends back on themselves, as in Rolnick's technique (1954), or by arranging the cut ends to overlap each other (Hanley, 1968)—as shown in Figure 10. But no less important is the avoidance of local bleeding and sperm leakage (Fernandes et al., 1968), which may lead to granuloma formation. Even if leakage does occur, and a granuloma forms, the chances that recanalisation will occur are obviously very significantly reduced if the cut ends of the vas point in opposite directions.

The general management of patients undergoing vasectomy for voluntary sterilisation has been described in detail elsewhere (Hanley, 1968) but certain points bear repetition, if only to

188

emphasise their importance. First and foremost, perhaps, is the fact that cases of this nature may have medico-legal consequences if there is failure to achieve sterilisation. There is a very real possibility that the operation might fail, and the operation itself is not without morbidity, and these facts need to be discussed fully with both the husband and the wife before an operation is undertaken. The need for repeated semen analyses in the post-operative period must also be stressed and during this time, of course, full contraceptive precautions must be taken. The operation should be carried out on an inpatient under general anæsthesia with adequate pre- and post-operative sedation. Hæmatoma formation, which usually develops within a few hours of operation, but is occasionally delayed (Stidolph, 1968), is to be avoided at all costs; if it does occur and is large, it is better to evacuate it in the theatre immediately than to attempt aspiration or allow it to absorb spontaneously. At operation the vasa should be explored through two separate 2 cm. scrotal incisions (Hanley, 1968), and small loops of vas should be isolated and divided as described above. It is a wise precaution to excise a small segment of each vas and submit it to the laboratory for histological confirmation of identity. Finally, it cannot be stressed too often that the patient should not be considered to be sterile until all spermatozoa have been ejaculated from that part of the system above the site of the ligature. This may take many months.

SUMMARY

In each of seven patients subjected to bilateral vasectomy for voluntary sterilisation there was subsequent spontaneous recanalisation of one vas. The pathological findings are discussed in detail, and the way in which recanalisation probably occurs, and the measures which need to be taken to prevent it, are described. The general management of patients is also discussed.

We are indebted to Mr Hickinbotham for allowing us to include his patient in our series, to the Editor of *The Lancet* for permission to reproduce Figures 8 and 10, and to the Medical Art Department at the Institute of Urology for the illustrations. We are particularly grateful to Mr G. R. Bryden, F.I.M.L.T., who prepared the many histological sections upon which this study was based.

REFERENCES

BUNGE, R. G. (1968). *J. Urol.*, **100**, 762.
FERNANDES, M., SHAH, K. N., and DRAPER, J. W. (1968). *J. Urol.*, **100**, 763.
GLASSY, F. J., and MOSTOFI, F. K. (1956). *Am. J. clin. Path.*, **26**, 1303.
HANLEY, H. G. (1968). *Lancet*, **2**, 207.
O'CONNOR, V. J. (1948). *J. Am. med. Ass.*, **136**, 162.
PHILLIPS, D. E. H. (1961). *Br. J. Urol.*, **33**, 448.
ROLNICK, H. C. (1954). *J. Urol.*, **72**, 915.
STIDOLPH, N. (1968). Personal communication.

VASOVASOSTOMY: IMPROVED MICROSURGICAL TECHNIQUE

MANUEL FERNANDES, KANU N. SHAH AND JOHN W. DRAPER

Vasectomy has become increasingly popular as a means of male sterilization.[1-4] Our interest was stimulated by our poor results in trying to restore continuity of the vasa for patients who have changed their minds. These frequent failures to restore continuity have mitigated against vasectomy even though it is simple to perform and is an effective means of promoting planned parenthood.[2, 4] The great variety of surgical procedures which have been suggested to accomplish a functioning vasovasostomy attest to the difficulty of the problem.[5-11]

By studying the techniques currently in use, we tried to establish a procedure which would be uniformly successful in experimental animals.[12-16]

This study was carried out with the help of a surgical microscope, special instruments adapted to its use and fine suture material. Two groups of young adult mongrel male dogs were used. The dogs weighed from 40 to 60 pounds.

Group 1 consisted of 12 dogs. After suitable skin preparation and draping, a small incision was made over the vas. The vas was divided about 1 cm. cranial to the convoluted part and anastomosed over a No. 32 stainless steel wire splint with 6 to 8 sutures of 7–zero black silk. The sutures were placed through the serosa and muscularis of the vas with the help of the operating microscope at 15 diameters. The wire splint was brought out through a small puncture wound in the vas, 1 cm. caudad to the anastomosis,[5] through the scrotum and anchored to the skin with a suture of 2–zero black silk. The splint remained in situ for 5 to 40 days except in 1 dog in which the splint was removed just after the anastomosis had been completed, as described by Roland.[6]

Group 2 consisted of 14 dogs in which 20 end-to-end vasovasostomies were carried out without the use of a splint (fig. 1). The artery of the vas could be dissected free of the vas for a distance of about 4 cm. Two small tourniquets were placed about the vas 2 cm. from the vasostomy and were held in place with small hemostats. These tourniquets provided a bloodless field for the anastomosis and prevented sperm from leaking out during the operation, thus reducing the chance of sperm granulomas.[2] A 1 cm. segment of the vas was excised and discarded. The

[1] Chaset, N.: Male sterilization. J. Urol., 87: 512–517, 1962.
[2] Schmidt, S. S.: Technics and complications of elective vasectomy. The role of spermatic granuloma in spontaneous recanalization. Fertil. Steril, 17: 167–482, 1966.
[3] Rieser, C.: Vasectomy: medical and legal aspects. J. Urol., 79: 138–144, 1958.
[4] Strode, J. E.: A technique of vasectomy for sterilization. J. Urol., 37: 733, 1937.
[5] O'Conor, V. J.: Anastomosis of the vas deferens after purposeful division for sterility. J. Urol., 59: 229–233, 1948.
[6] Roland, S. I.: Splinted and non-splinted vasovasostomy. A review of the literature and a report of nine new cases. Fertil. Steril., 12: 191–195, 1961.
[7] Massey, B. D. and Nation, E. F.: Vas deferens anastomosis: a report of four consecutive successful cases. J. Urol., 61: 391–395, 1949.
[8] Freiberg, H. B. and Lepsky, H. O.: Restoration of the continuity of the vas deferens eight years after bilateral vasectomy. J. Urol., 41: 934, 1939.
[9] Dorsey, J. W.: Anastomosis of the vas deferens to correct post-vasectomy sterility. J. Urol., 70: 515–519, 1953.
[10] Cameron, C. S.: Anastomosis of the vas deferens. J.A.M.A., 127: 1119–1120, 1945.
[11] Waller, J. I. and Turner, T. A.: Anastomosis of the vas after vasectomy. J. Urol., 88: 409–410, 1962.
[12] Schmidt, S. S.: Anastomosis of the vas deferens: an experimental study. II. Successes and failures in experimental anastomosis. J. Urol., 81: 203–205, 1959.
[13] Schmidt, S. S.: Anastomosis of the vas deferens: an experimental study. I. J. Urol., 75: 300–303, 1956.
[14] Magoss, I., Persky, L., Austen, G., Jr. and Orbison, L.: The effect of cortisone on experimental vasovasostomy. J. Urol., 78: 78–81, 1957.
[15] Schmidt, S. S.: Anastomosis of the vas deferens: an experimental study. III. Dilatation of the vas following obstruction. J. Urol., 81: 205–208, 1959.
[16] Schmidt, S. S.: Anastomosis of the vas deferens: an experimental study. IV, The use of fine polyethylene tubing as a splint. J. Urol., 85: 838–841, 1961.

190

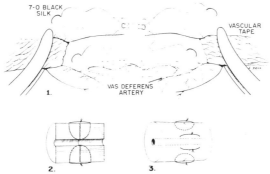

FIG. 1. Microvasovasostomy without splint

TABLE 1. *Microsurgical technique with No. 32 wire splint*

Vasovasostomy	No. Cases	No. Anastomosis	Failure	Success
Splint *out* after operation	1	1	1	0
Splint *out* after 5 days	9	9	7	2
Splint *in* for 6 weeks	2	2	2	0
Total	12	12	10	2

remaining unspatulated ends were approximated by placing a suture of 7–zero black silk with a swedged, curved ophthalmic needle on each end through the lumen and out through the wall of the vas at 12 and 6 o'clock. Thus, the lumen of the vas was aligned without the aid of a splint. Then 2 to 4 additional sutures were placed equidistally about the cut edge, passing the needle through the serosa and muscularis only. These sutures effectively provided good approximation and prevented sperm leakage. A silver clip was secured to one of the sutures of the anastomosis to demonstrate the site by x-ray. The 2 tourniquets were then removed and slight bleeding was noted, indicating satisfactory blood supply. The inguinal incision was closed using 3–zero chromic catgut.

Six weeks postoperatively vasograms were performed to demonstrate patency of the vas and anastomosis. This procedure was carried out by exposing the vas in its convoluted portion and, through a small puncture wound, a No. 25 hypodermic needle was inserted toward the anasto-

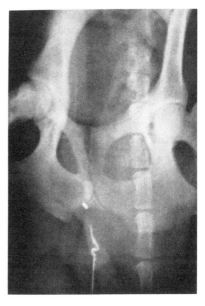

FIG. 2. Vasogram 6 weeks after vasovasostomy demonstrates obstructed lumen at exit site of splint. Anastomosis site is marked with silver clip.

mosis. After 1 cc hypaque 50 per cent was injected, films were taken.

Three to 6 months later orchiectomy with removal of the entire vas was performed. Again, patency of the fresh specimen was determined by injecting saline solution into the lumen of the

191

vas through a No. 25 needle. The specimens were then placed in formalin for histological sections.

RESULTS

Nine of 12 animals in group 1 pulled out the wire splint between 1 to 6 weeks postoperatively (table 1). Seven of the 9 animals were found to be failures with obstruction of the lumen at the exit site of the splint caudad to the anastomosis (fig. 2). The remaining 2 anastomoses were considered successes with normal looking vasograms.

Two of the 12 dogs were found to have the wire splint in place 6 weeks postoperatively. The splints were removed and a vasogram was made using the technique previously described. To our surprise, in both cases obstruction of the lumen was found. In one dog the obstruction was at the site where the splint was brought out, approximately 1 cm. caudad to the anastomosis, (marked with a silver slip) and in the other dog obstruction was found approximately 2 to 3 cm. cranial to the anastomosis in the area of the vas which had been splinted for 6 weeks (figs. 3 to 4). In both cases gross and microscopic examination revealed a patent anastomosis. The splint was

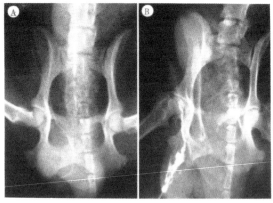

FIG. 3. Dog 2. *A*, plain film demonstrates No. 32 wire splint within vas lumen 6 weeks after vaso-vasostomy. *B*, vasogram immediately after removal of splint demonstrates obstructed vas lumen 2 to 3 cm. cranial to anastomosis.

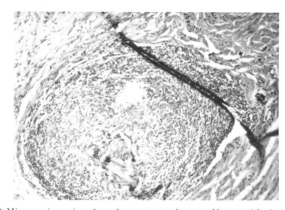

FIG. 4. Dog 2. Microscopic section of vas demonstrates obstructed lumen with giant cells and chronic inflammatory cells (foreign body reaction).

192

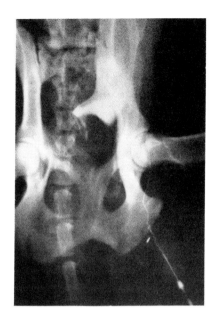

removed immediately after the anastomosis was accomplished in 1 dog; in this case obstruction of the lumen was noted at the site of the anastomosis.

In our second group of animals with vasovasos-

TABLE 2. *Improved microsurgical technique without splints*

Vasovasostomy	No. Cases	No. Anastomosis	Failure	Success
Unilateral	8	8	0	8
Bilateral	6	12	1	11
Total	14	20	1	19

tomy without a splint, the vasogram at 6 weeks (fig. 5) and the injection of saline solution of the fresh specimen after 6 months revealed patency with excellent morphological and functional repair in 19 of 20 anastomoses (table 2). Vasotomy 6 months after the anastomosis revealed equal numbers of motile sperm in the lumen of the vas on both sides of the anastomosis.

At the time of removal of the specimen, more fibrosis and scar tissue were noted in dogs in which a splint had been used.

CONCLUSION

Twelve anastomoses carried out with the aid of a No. 32 wire splint resulted in 10 failures. Failure was usually caused by scarring at the exit of the splint from the lumen of the vas.

The anastomosis with similar microsurgical technique without splinting was successful in 19 of 20 anastomoses. Success was demonstrated by vasograms, saline injection of the removed vasa, microscopic sections and the presence of sperm having passed through the anastomosis.

Vasovasostomy — A Simplified Technique

Edward E. Steinhardt M.D.

No reports of significance regarding reunion of the vas deferens after an intentional ligation appeared in the literature until 1948. O'Conor then reported on 14 patients who underwent bilateral reunion with successful results in 9.[1] His criteria for success were repeated counts of spermatozoa above 20 million per cc with normal morphology and motility.[2] He had a 2 to 15 year followup. A questionnaire sent to 1,240 urologists at the time showed 420 operations performed with a success rate of 35 to 40%. Success was shown by the appearance of spermatozoa in the semen.

O'Conor later reported 24 more vasovasostomies with a success rate of 43%.[3] His technique was excision of the scarred vas, and end to end anastomosis using silkworm gut as a splint. This splint was removed in 6 to 10 days.

Experimental work by Schmidt[4] showed that successful results were best obtained by end to end anastomosis, gentle handling of tissues, prophylactic antibiotics, internal splinting for 10 days and fine sutures. His results were 50% successful in dogs, using an internal splint of 3-0 nylon. Failures were due mostly to spermatic granulomata, although improper alignment, separation, fibrosis, and infection were contributing factors.[5] He later improved his technique with a No. 2 F polyethylene tubing as a splint which was brought through the wall of the vas at a location 1 cm distal to the anastomosis.[6] The tubing was then fixed to the skin where it drained for 10 days and then was removed. In all 10 dogs, the anastomosis remained patent.

Various urologists using an internal splint and fine sutures have reported successful human vasovasostomies in from 77 to 88% of patients[7-10] Goodwin[11] felt that the rate of success with skillful technique could be 90%. Moon and Bunge[12] reported that in their experience nonsplinted anastomoses had a 12% superiority over the splinted technique in their 11 dogs, and the splints went through the proximal and distal walls of the vas. Phadke and Phadke[13] reported on 76 patients with 83% successful appearance of spermatozoa. For 55% pregnancy resulted in their mates. The Phadkes used meticulous technique, an internal splint for eight days, prophylactic antibiotics, and bed rest for one week. Fernandes et al[14] recently described a microsurgical technique for vasavasostomy in dogs, in which splinted and nonsplinted anastomoses were used. In their hands the nonsplinted technique was far superior.

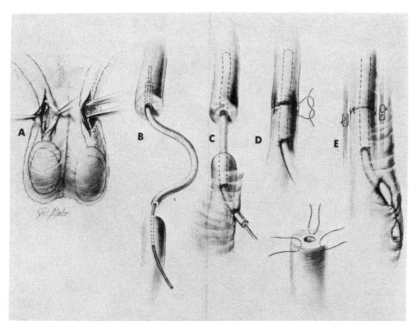

Figure 1

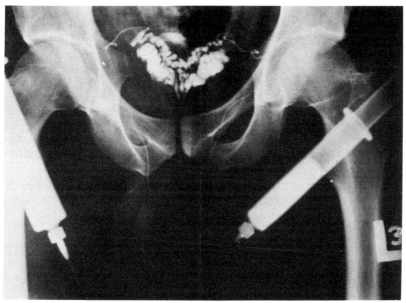

Figure 2A
Injection of 1cc 50% Hypaque in proximal vas.

195

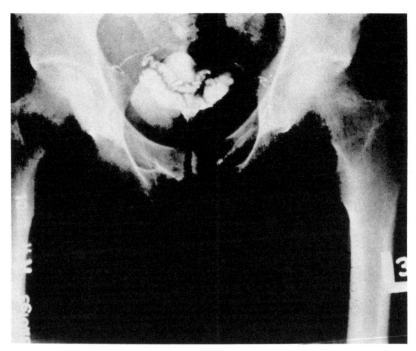

Figure 2B
Appearance of radioopaque medium in bladder showing patency.

Personal Technique

The technique we employ was developed for its simplicity and adaptability, and attempts to incorporate the best of the preceding experiences. Fine instruments are used with either general or spinal anesthesia. A high scrotal incision is made and the scarred ends of the vas are excised (Fig. 1A). The proximal vas will show a milky secretion. A dilute indigo carmine solution can be injected easily into the distal vas, and will appear in the bladder. Having established patency, a readily available polyethylene catheter* is then threaded over a No. 28 wire. Using the projecting end of the wire for an obturator, the tubing is passed several cms into the distal vas. The wire is passed up the proximal vas for 1 cm and pushed through the wall, and fixed to the skin with suture and aeroplast spray (Fig. 1B & C).

An end to end anastomosis is done using three sutures of 6-0 dermalon through the wall of the vas avoiding the lumen (Fig. 1C). The tissues around the vas are approximated with 6-0 dermalon to prevent stress on the anastomsis. (Fig. 1D and E). The patient is given tetracycline for 10 days postoperatively, is out of bed the first postoperative day, and goes home on the second postoperative day, wearing a scrotal support. When he returns on the tenth postoperative day, the splint is removed, after which he is advised to resume intercourse. Periodic semen analyses are done.

---

*B.D. tubing (VX020).

196

Representative Patient

R.L.B., #1340193-0, was a 28-year-old white factory worker who had had a bilateral partial vasectomy at age 21 for socio-economic reasons (he had three children in this first marriage). He then remarried and desired further children. His examination showed bilateral upper scrotal scars and his semen showed the absence of sperm. In August, 1968, he underwent a bilateral vasovasostomy using an internal polyethylene splint. His postoperative course was uneventful and he went home on his second postoperative day. Splints were removed on the tenth postoperative day. A seminal vesiculogram (Figures 2A and 2B) showed patency of the anastomosis. He resumed intercourse, and a sperm count three weeks later was 20 million, with normal appearance and motility. On a subsequent visit, he stated that his wife was pregnant.

One final word — Vasovasostomy is much easier to accomplish if the previous sterilization procedure had been done with consideration given to the possibility that the patient may have a future change of plans. A high scrotal incision over the straight portion of the vas should be used. The vas should be lightly fulgurated, and one end should be covered with a sheath of tissue.[15]

REFERENCES

1. O'Conor, V.J.: Anastomosis of vas deferens after purposeful division for sterility, *JAMA* 136:162-3, Jan 17, 1948.

2. O'Conor, V.J.: Mechanical aspects and surgical management of sterility in men, *JAMA* 153:532-4, Oct 10, 1953.

3. O'Conor, V.J.: Mechanical aspects of surgical correction of male sterility, *Fertil Steril* 4:439-55, Nov-Dec 1953.

4. Schmidt, S.S.: Anastomosis of the vas deferens: an experimental study, *J Urol* 75:300-3, Feb 1956.

5. Schmidt, S.S.: Anastomosis of the vas deferens: an experimental study. II and III, *J Urol* 81:203-8, Jan 1959.

6. Schmidt, S.S.: Anastomosis of the vas deferens: an experimental study. IV. The use of fine polyethylene tubing as a splint, *J Urol* 85:838-41, May 1961.

7. Phadke, G.M.: Re-anastomosis of the vas deferens, *J Indian Med Ass* 36:386-90, May 1, 1961.

8. Roland, S.I.: Splinted and non-splinted vasovasostomy, *Fertil Steril* 12:191-5, Mar-Apr 1961.

9. Dorsey, J.W.: Surgical correction of postvasectomy sterility, *J Int Coll Surg* 27:453-6, Apr 1957.

10. Jhaver, P.S.: *J Family Welfare* 9:57, 1962.

11. Brewer, H.: Reversibility following sterilization by vasectomy, *Eugen Rev* 56:147-50, Oct 1964.

12. Moon, K.H., and Bunge, R.G.: Splinted and nonsplinted vasovasostomy: experimental study, *Invest Urol* 5:155-60, Sept 1967.

13. Phadke, G.M., and Phadke, A.G.: Experiences in the re-anastomosis of the vas deferens, *J Urol* 97:888-90, May 1967.

14. Fernandes, M.; Shah, K.N.; and Draper, J.H.: Vasovasostomy: improved micro-surgical technique, *J Urol* 100:763-6, Dec 1968.

15. Schmidt, S.S.: Vasectomy: indications, technic and reversibility, *Fertil Steril* 19:192-6, Mar-Apr 1968.

SPLINTED AND NONSPLINTED VASOVASOSTOMY: EXPERIMENTAL STUDY

K. H. Moon and R. G. Bunge

Vasectomy has become a popular procedure for establishment of permanent sterility. However, requests for restoration of fertility potential appear from time to time by patients who have remarried. There is belief in some quarters that a positive, highly successful method of anastomosis would encourage more fathers to accept vasectomy.

Since the first anastomosis of the ductus deferens was attempted by Martin in 1902, successful operations have been carried out by many surgeons with many different techniques (1–5). It is, however, a controversial matter whether a splint should be used to obtain the best possible results. It was to this problem we addressed ourselves.

MATERIALS AND METHODS

Eleven adult male dogs varying from 13 to 18 kg in weight were used. In each dog, after severance of the duct, a no. 3 nylon splint was employed on the right and none on the left to perform the anastomosis. In 2 of the 11 dogs, modification was necessary because of nondescent of the left testis in one, and a surgical accident, preventing anastomosis, on the right in the other.

Under intravenous Nembutal anesthesia, and after the usual skin preparation, both ducts were exposed through a high midscrotal incision. A 2-cm segment of each duct was then dissected free at a point 2 cm above the upper pole of the epididymis and then severed (Fig. 1). On the left side a no. 23 hypodermic needle was inserted into the distal lumen for a distance of 1 cm and then directed through the wall (Fig. 1B).

A similar procedure was performed on the proximal segment (Fig. 1C), but here, in addition, a second needle was guided through the wall and out the lumen by the first needle (Fig. 1D). A no. 3 nylon thread was directed through the inserted needles, which were then removed (Fig. 1E), leaving the segments of the duct suspended upon a sling (Fig. 1F). Approximation of the ends was

This study was supported by Grant M66.075 from the Population Council, Inc., Rockefeller Institute, New York, New York.

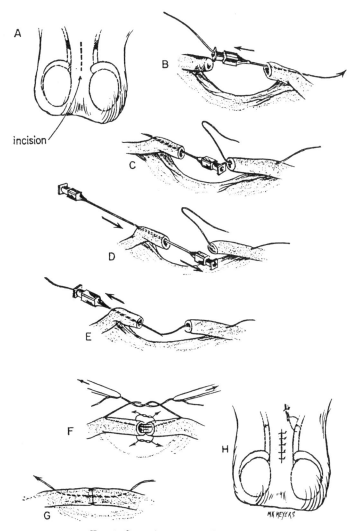

FIG. 1. Steps in vasovasostomy

accomplished by three interrupted no. 6 silk sutures placed equidistantly around the circumference of the line of approximation (Fig. 1G). The suspending nylon suture was then removed. The right severed duct was similarly joined, but the free ends of the nylon suture were loosely tied together, brought out to the skin, and anchored to the upper end of the surgical scrotal wound (Fig. 1H).

Closure of the skin edges was obtained with interrupted no. 3 silk sutures (Fig. 1H). The splint was removed 10 to 14 days postoperatively. The scrotal contents were removed 17 to 24 days postoperatively. The anastomosed duct was dissected free beyond both needle puncture sites and examined grossly

199

and microscopically. Patency was determined visually by injection of indigo carmine into the lumen and radiographically by injection of 70 per cent Hypaque.

RESULTS

A total of 11 anastomoses was done by the nonsplint method (Table 1), and the patency was established in 9 of them for a success rate of 82 per cent. Two of the failure cases, no. 6 and 7, revealed that no. 6 showed a moderate degree of epididymoorchitis postoperatively, which might have been the cause of the failure. The second case, no. 7, showed that at the site of anastomosis there was delayed healing and that the severed ends were easily separated. Grossly there was very slight granulation tissue around the site in every case. Histologic studies showed that in every patent duct there was no significant inflammatory tissue reaction at the anastomotic site (Fig. 2A). The lesion areas of needle punctures likewise showed no tissue reaction.

A total of ten anastomoses was attempted by splinted method (Table 1), and the patency was 70 per cent. Grossly there was a significant amount of local tissue reaction around the anastomotic site, and microscopically there was no significant reaction within the wall at the anastomotic site (Fig. 2B). Generally granulation tissue formed around the anastomotic site of the splinted side, whereas it was remarkably absent in the nonsplinted cases.

DISCUSSION

In 1948, O'Conor (6), from a questionnaire mailed to United States urologists, reported a successful recanalization of the ductus deferens after reanasto-

TABLE 1. *Comparative study of nonsplint and splint method*

Dog No.	Splint		Nonsplint	
	Patency	L.T.R.*	Patency	L.T.R.
1	†		+	Minimum
2	+	Marked	+	Minimum
3	+	Marked	+	Minimum
4	+	Minimum	+	Minimum
5	+	Minimum	+	Minimum
6	−	Marked	−	Marked
7	−	Marked	−	Marked
8	+	Marked	+	Minimum
9	+	Marked	+	Minimum
10	+	Marked	+	Minimum
11	−	Marked	+	Minimum
Patency	7		9	
Total cases	10		11	
Percentage of success	70		82	

* Local tissue reaction.
† Surgery not attempted.

200

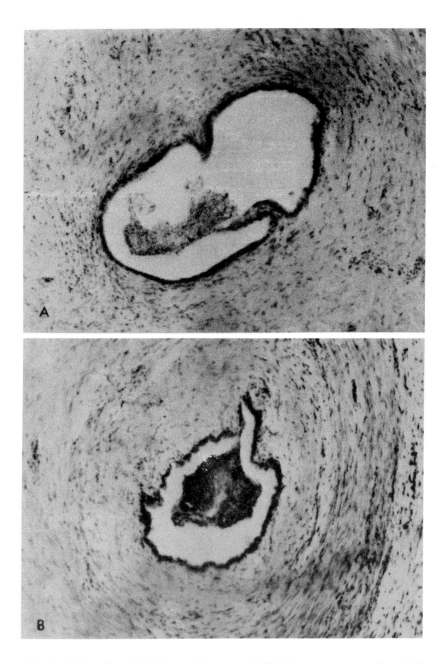

FIG. 2. *A*, Nonsplinted left ductus deferens, no. 9. The lumen was patent. No significant tissue reaction was found in the wall. Hematoxylin and eosin, ×200. *B*, Splinted, right ductus deferens, no. 10. The lumen was patent. No significant tissue reaction was found in the wall. Hematoxylin and eosin, ×200.

201

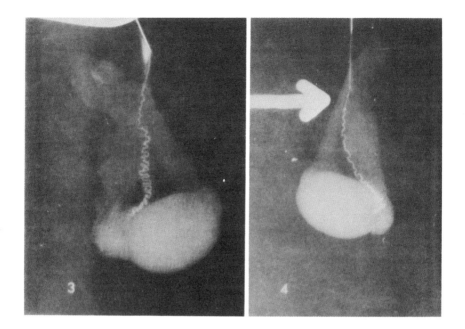

FIG. 3. Epididymovasography right splinted, no. 10. The lumen was patent
FIG. 4. Epididymovasography left nonsplinted, no. 9. The lumen was patent

mosis in approximately 45.5 per cent. Other reports were 35 to 40 per cent by Mauritzen (7), 38 per cent by Rosenbloom (8), 75 per cent by Humphreys and Hotchkiss (9), 58 per cent by Hagner (10), and 30 per cent by Michelson (11). In animal experiments, Schmidt (12) reported the operation was successful in 50 per cent. Reporting investigators used splints of plain and chromic catgut, silk, horse hair, silver wire, ureteral catheter, nylon, and polyethylene tubes. However, there is no conclusive data that would indicate the material best suited for splinting. Very few attempts have been made to evaluate the nonsplint method in reviewing the literature available to us. Handly (13) reported on the nonsplinted method with a highly successful result. Recently Roland (14) reported seven successful bilateral anastomoses in nine patients with 77 per cent success.

Surveying our own data of nonsplint versus splint methods in dogs, we have concluded that the nonsplint method appears to be superior for the following reasons:

1) Grossly and histologically the nonsplinted site had remarkably less tissue reaction than the splinted site.

2) An avenue of infection along the splint is removed by the absence of such a device.

3) Less postoperative care was required, and loss of the splint prematurely was avoided.

4) The nonsplint procedure is less complicated, affords a good rate of patency, and avoids tissue aggravation by the splint.

Acknowledgments. The authors gratefully acknowledge the technical help of Charles Kingsbury.

REFERENCES

1. Waller, J. I., and Turner, T. A.: Anastomosis of the vas after vasectomy. J. Urol., *88:* 409, 1962.
2. Dorsey, J. W.: Anastomosis of vas deferens to correct post-vasectomy sterility. J. Urol., *70:* 515, 1953.
3. O'Conor, V. J.: Mechanical aspects and surgical management of sterility in men. J.A.M.A., *153:* 532, 1953.
4. Busse, E.: Reunion of vas deferens after surgical sterilization. Deutsch. Gesundh., *5:* 530, 1950.
5. Massey, B. D., and Nation, E. F.: Vas deferens anastomosis: report of four consecutive successful cases. J. Urol., *61:* 391, 1949.
6. O'Conor, V. J.: Anastomosis operations on the vas deferens after purposeful division for sterility. J.A.M.A., *136:* 162, 1948.
7. Mauritzen, K.: Anastomotic operations on the vas deferens. Acta Chir. Scand., *102:* 457, 1952.
8. Rosenbloom, D.: Reversal of sterility due to vasectomy. Fertil. Steril., *7:* 540, 1956.
9. Humphreys, G. A., and Hotchkiss, R. S.: Vasoepididymal anastomosis. J. Urol., *42:* 815, 1939.
10. Hagner, F. R.: Sterility in the male. Surg. Gynec. Obstet., *52:* 330, 1931.
11. Michelson, L.: Vasoepididymal anastomosis by producing a permanent fistula with use of stainless steel wire. Surg. Gynec. Obstet., *82:* 327, 1946.
12. Schmidt, S. S.: Anastomosis of the vas deferens: an experimental study. II. Successes and failures in experimental anastomosis. J. Urol., *81:* 203, 1959.
13. Handly, R. S.: Reconstruction of vas deferens after operation for sterilization. Arch. Middlesex Hosp., *1:* 74, 1951.
14. Roland, S. I.: Splinted and non-splinted vasovasostomy. Fertil. Steril., *12:* 191, 1961.

BILATERAL SPONTANEOUS REANASTOMOSIS OF THE DUCTUS DEFERENS

R. G. BUNGE

Spontaneous reanastomosis of the surgically interrupted ductus deferens is a well-documented fact. Such spontaneity of Mother Nature engenders marital discord and wild, spousal conjectures, both of which are abated by a semen analysis. However, the full fury now turns on the vasectomist. The surgeon should carefully explain this possibility to his patient and should have a written operative consent signed by both husband and wife in which there is a statement acknowledging this complication by both signatories.

CASE REPORT

R. D. A., a 33-year-old white man, presented himself for fertility investigation. Although 6 years previously the patient had had a bilateral vasectomy, his wife had become pregnant several months ago. The patient related that the pregnancy had terminated in a spontaneous miscarriage and that he and his wife wished to avoid another such experience. He had no surgical facts relating to the vasectomy.

No abnormalities were discovered by the physical examination. A semenogram showed, after 30 days of continence, a volume of 0.8 ml., normal liquefaction, a count of 45 million per ml. viability of 65 per cent (35 per cent abnormal forms) and fair sperm motility.

Bilateral exploration of the scrotal contents revealed a small, scarred nodule, approximately 0.5 cm. in diameter, on the right side; the nodule and a segment of the ductus deferens on either side of the nodule were removed. On the left, no nodule could be found and a 5 cm. segment of the duct was removed.

Radiographs of the specimens, made by injecting radiopaque liquid, show continuity of both ducts, the one on the right having a sperm granuloma (fig. 1). Microscopic examination of the nodule confirmed the impression of a sperm granuloma (fig. 2). Unfortunately the left specimen was lost before microscopic examination could be performed.

SUMMARY

Spontaneous reanastomosis of the ductus deferens, one with a sperm granuloma, has been demonstrated following vasectomies 6 years before.

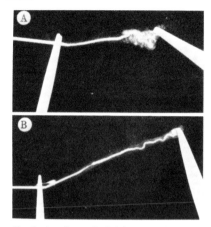

FIG. 1. *A*, radiograph of right surgical specimen after injection with liquid radiopaque material shows continuity of ductus deferens and extravasation into structure identified as sperm granuloma. *B*, radiograph of left surgical specimen shows continuity of ductus deferens in mid-portion. Proximal end of duct is on right.

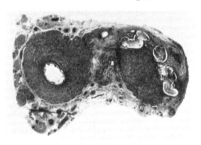

FIG. 2. Low power photomicrograph of right surgical specimen containing scarred nodule. Flushed-out empty ductus deferens is on left and accumulations of spermatozoa and granulomatous tissue are on right.

A SIMPLE TECHNIQUE OF RE-ANASTOMOSIS AFTER VASECTOMY

By K. C. Mehta, M.S., and P. S. Ramani, M.S.

The wider use of vasectomy as one of the methods of family planning is likely to bring in its wake an increasing demand for re-anastomosis, though in only a small percentage of individuals.

This paper is based on an experience of 26 restorative operations. In the first 3 cases end-to-end anastomosis of the vas (O'Conor, 1948), was carried out, but we were soon convinced that side-to-side anastomosis would be better (6 cases) in preventing post-operative stenosis. Further, during re-operation on a failed case from our initial series, we found extensive fibrosis replacing the vas at the site of anastomosis. We believed that this was due to avascular necrosis of the vas

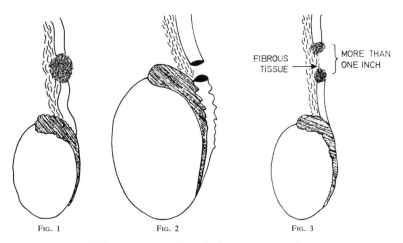

FIG. 1   FIG. 2   FIG. 3

Different appearances of cut ends of vas as seen at operation.

as a result of interference of blood supply due to excessive mobilisation. Like the ureter, a mobilised vas, when divided transversely undergoes avascular necrosis (Swinney and Hammersley, 1963).

Thus the present technique of side-to-side anastomosis without mobilisation of the vas was evolved and used in 17 consecutive cases.

Reasons for Re-anastomosis.—The indications for re-anastomosis were remarriage, death of a male child or children, desire to have more children and for psychological reasons. In this series vasectomy was performed on 5 patients who had no children, 2 of whom were not even married. In 2 patients there had been accidental injury to the vas during operations for hydrocele and inguinal hernia. Three patients were re-operated on for failure of the initial re-anastomosis. The interval between vasectomy and re-anastomosis varied from 3 months to 4 years.

Pre-operative Evaluation.—Pre-operative evaluation of the scar, the spermatic cord, the vas, the epididymes and testes was helpful in planning the operation. There was no dilatation of the

205

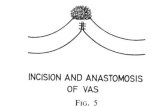

INCISION AND ANASTOMOSIS
OF VAS

Fig. 4   Fig. 5

Fig. 4.—Method of incision of proximal and distal ends of vas. For details see text.

Fig. 5.—Anastomosis of the two incised ends.

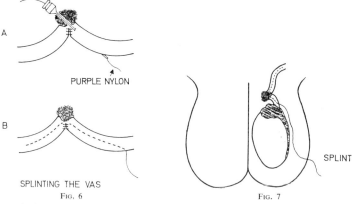

A

PURPLE NYLON

B

SPLINT

SPLINTING THE VAS

Fig. 6   Fig. 7

Fig. 6.—A and B, Method of splinting the vas with purple nylon. The splint is threaded into the vas through the lumen of a syringe needle.

Fig. 7.—Splint in position at the end of the operation.

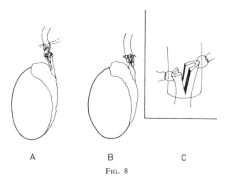

A   B   C

Fig. 8

A, B and C, Methods of anastomosis when vasectomy is performed near the narrow convoluted part of the vas. For details see text. Figure 8, C is a magnified view showing details of anastomosis.

proximal vas (Phadke and Phadke, 1967) but in the majority the epididymes showed enlargement. The testes did not show any variation from the normal except for partial atrophy on one side in 2 patients in whom the anastomosis had been attempted elsewhere. The different appearances of the cut ends of the vas as seen at operation are shown in Figures 1, 2 and 3.

Technique of Operation.—Fourteen patients were operated on under spinal anæsthesia and the remaining 3 under general anæsthesia. The average time taken for operation was 75 minutes. A vertical upper scrotal 2-inch long incision is made. An upward extension of this incision to the external inguinal ring is occasionally necessary. The cord is delivered and the cut ends of the vas surrounded by a small fibrous mass are identified. Mobilisation of the vas either from the cord or from the fibrous mass is unnecessary as this is associated with risk of injury to its blood supply and that of the testes. The normal-looking vas just proximal and distal to the fibrous mass is incised transversely until the lumen is entered, care being taken not to transect the vas completely. A 24 gauge B.D. needle is passed into the lumen and brought out through the wall about 3 mm. away. A fine pointed knife is engaged in the bevel of the needle and the vas is incised longitudinally as the needle is withdrawn (Fig. 4).

If the operation is done less than a year after vasectomy milky fluid oozes out through the proximal end. This fluid must be washed away with normal saline to prevent formation of a sperm granuloma (Lyons et al., 1967). Normal saline, 2-3 ml., is injected into the distal cut end to ascertain its patency.

The 2 incised ends are anastomosed side-to-side with 2-3 posterior and 2-3 anterior interrupted stitches (Fig. 5). These stitches are passed through partial thickness of the wall without entering the lumen and the knots are tied on the outer side. A purple nylon splint (Campbell, 1963) is introduced before inserting the anterior stitches (Fig. 6). Nylon, 5/0, on a atraumatic needle is used for anastomosis. One or two stay stitches are taken through the soft tissues around the vas. The cord is replaced, the end of the nylon splint is brought out through the scrotal wall and the incision is closed in layers (Fig. 7).

When vasectomy has been performed near the narrow convoluted part of the vas, a new technique is used instead of standard epididymovasostomy. The cut ends are separated from the fibrous mass carefully without extensive mobilisation. The proximal cut end is incised on each side longitudinally for a distance of about 2 mm., thus creating 2 split flaps. Then the 2 split ends are drawn into the lumen of the distal vas. A stitch is placed at the edge of each split flap. Each end of this stitch is brought out through the wall of the distal vas at a distance of about 2 mm. and a knot is tied on the outer side (Fig. 8, A, B and C). This technique was used unilaterally on 3 occasions. Since 2 of these 3 patients had nearly normal semen analysis following the operation the technique is presumed to be successful.

Post-operative Mamagement.—Complete rest in bed is advised for a week. The nylon splint is removed along with the skin stitches on the seventh day. Broad spectrum antibiotics and anti-inflammatory agents, indomethacine (Indocid-M.S.D.) or oxyphenbutazone (Tanderil-Geigy) are administered routinely. Prednisolone (30 mg. daily) is given orally for a week after healing of the wound. Semen analysis is carried out after 3 weeks and repeated when necessary.

Results.—The appearance of spermatozoa in the semen suggests a successful result, though the count may not return to normal for 3 to 6 months. If there are no sperms after 3 months the operation is considered to be a failure. In our experience, none of the failures ever showed spermatozoa after 3 months. Of the last 17 operations only 2 failed.

CONCLUSIONS

Vasectomy is reversible in the majority, if anastomosis is carried out meticulously. The reasons for failure are infection, hæmatoma, injury to the blood supply of the vas and testis,

207

blocked lumen and faulty technique. Avascular necrosis of the vas due to extensive mobilisation leading to fibrosis is in our opinion a major cause of failure.

Fibrosis, hæmatoma and injury to the blood supply of the vas and testis can all be prevented by the technique described here.

We thank the Dean, T.N. Medical College, for permission to use the records of some of the patients.

Addendum:—Since the submission of this article for publication, 5 more side-to-side anastomoses of the vas have been carried out, with success in all.

REFERENCES

CAMPBELL, M. F. (1963). " Urology ", Vol. 1, p. 678. Philadelphia: Saunders.

GLASSY, F. J. and MOSTOFI, F. K. (1956). Spermatic granuloma of epididymis. *American Journal of Clinical Pathology*, **26**, 1303-1313.

LYONS, R. C., PETRE, J. H. and CHUL NAM LEE (1967). Spermatic granuloma of epididymis. *Journal of Urology*, **97**, 320-323.

O'CONOR, V. J. (1948). Anastomosis of vas deferens after purposeful division for sterility. *Journal of the American Medical Association*, **136**, 162-163.

PHADKE, G. M. and PHADKE, A. G. (1967). Experiences in reanastomosis of vas deferens. *Journal of Urology*, **97**, 888-890.

SCHMIDT, S. S. (1956). Anastomosis of vas deferens. An experimental study. *Journal of Urology*, **75**, 300-304.

SUNDERASIVARAO, D. (1955). Spermatozoal granuloma of epididymis. *Journal of Pathology and Bacteriology*, **69**, 324-326.

SWINNEY, J. and HAMMERSLEY, D. P. (1963). " A Handbook of Operative Urological Surgery ", p. 67. Edinburgh: Livingstone.

Veterinary Vasectomy

Gonadal and Extragonadal Sperm Reserves after Unilateral Vasoligation in Rabbits

K. L. MACMILLAN, Ph.D., C. DESJARDINS, Ph.D.,
K. T. KIRTON, Ph.D., and H. D. HAFS, Ph.D.

THE FATE OF SPERMATOGENESIS after vasoligation has been a subject of considerable controversy. Bouin and Ancel pointed out the disparity of results of others with different species and observed that vasoligation resulted in degeneration of guinea-pig spermiogenic tissue. Steinach reported that vasectomy in rabbits induced an initial decline in spermatogenesis, but that partial recovery occurred 3 weeks later. Moore and Quick considered that their results in rabbits did not support either of these conclusions: they suggested that vasectomy reduced spermatogenesis only if the surgery altered the normal scrotal position of the testis. All the conclusions in these early reports were based on testicular histologic evidence.

Amann estimated daily sperm production in vasectomized bulls and concluded that unilateral vasectomy did not alter sperm production in the testes on either side. His data led to the suggestion that the main site of bull sperm resorption was the cauda epididymidis. This is in agreement with Albert's proposal that resorption in fluid and sperm from the epididymis would prevent obstructive necrosis of the testis after vasoligation.

The present experiment was designed to determine the effects of unilateral vasoligation on the gonadal and extragonadal sperm reserves of rabbits, and to determine whether the epididymis of this species is capable of resorbing sperm.

MATERIAL AND METHODS

Under Surital anesthesia, a scrotal incision was made and the left deferent duct was ligated, excluding blood vessels, within 3 mm. of the epididymis in each of 25 sexually mature rabbits. The rabbits were regularly examined throughout the experimental period to be certain that the testis remained in the scrotum without adhesions.

At 1, 2, 3, 4, and 5 weeks after vasoligation, 5 rabbits were castrated. The testicular parenchymal tissue was weighed and homogenized in 50 ml. of 0.85% saline for 2 min. The caput-corpus and cauda epididymides were weighed and homogenized in 25 ml. and 50 ml. saline, respectively. Sperm numbers were determined hemacytometrically by previously reported procedures.[5]

Five rabbits were castrated as 0-day controls at the outset of the experiment and 10 rabbits were subjected to the entire surgical procedure except for the actual ligation. Five of the latter 10 rabbits were castrated 1 week and 5 were castrated 2 weeks later as sham-operated controls. The total number of sperm per testicular or epididymidal sample was calculated from the average of 4 hemacytometric counts, 2 made independently by each of 2 people.

Analyses of variance compared differences between data obtained on the ligated left side and the unligated right side in the 25 rabbits which had been subjected to unilateral ligation. Orthogonal polynomial analyses were used to determine the nature of response trends with interval of vasoligation.

Data from the control rabbits were analyzed to determine whether differences existed between left and right sides of the reproductive tract. Similar analyses of the data from the 1-week and 2-week sham-operated rabbits tested whether the surgery, apart from ligation, affected gonadal and extragonadal sperm reserves.

RESULTS

Average weights for the right (control) and left (ligated) sides for testes and caput-corpus and cauda epididymides in each group of rabbits are presented in Table 1. Although ligation of the left deferent duct caused a small decline in average weight of left testes ($p < 0.05$), the weight trends with duration of ligation within right or left sides were not significant. Neither did ligation affect significantly the average weight of the caput-corpus epididymides, but the weekly weight averages for both the ligated and normal sides showed a linear increase with duration of vasoligation ($p < 0.05$). The most dramatic effect of ligation was on cauda epididymides, which were significantly heavier on the ligated side ($p < 0.01$) where average weight increased linearly with duration of vasoligation ($p < 0.001$).

Averages for total and concentration of testicular sperm (Table 2) re-

211

TABLE 1. Weights of Testes, Caput-Corpus Epididymides, and Cauda Epididymides after Unilateral Vasoligation (gm.)

Duration of ligation (wk.)	Testis		Epididymis			
			Caput-corpus		Cauda	
	Normal	Ligated	Normal	Ligated	Normal	Ligated
0	1.00	1.02	0.15	0.15	0.25	0.25
1	0.97	0.88	0.15	0.15	0.27	0.32
2	1.39	0.88	0.19	0.22	0.32	0.43
3	1.53	1.32	0.22	0.22	0.34	0.56
4	1.34	1.38	0.21	0.23	0.32	0.61
5	1.20	1.07	0.20	0.22	0.32	0.53

TABLE 2. Concentration of Testicular Sperm and Total Testicular Sperm after Unilateral Vasoligation (Mean ± S.E.)

Duration of ligation (wk.)	Concentration ($\times 10^7$/gm.)		Total ($\times 10^7$/testis)	
	Normal	Ligated	Normal	Ligated
0	8.6 ± 0.8	8.5 ± 0.4	8.5 ± 0.9	8.7 ± 1.1
1	8.4 ± 0.9	5.8 ± 1.4	8.4 ± 2.0	5.9 ± 1.8
2	9.4 ± 0.8	3.3 ± 1.8	13.4 ± 2.8	4.5 ± 2.7
3	7.9 ± 0.5	6.0 ± 1.5	12.3 ± 2.1	9.5 ± 2.9
4	9.2 ± 0.6	7.2 ± 0.9	12.4 ± 1.0	9.9 ± 1.3
5	8.6 ± 0.4	6.5 ± 1.7	10.1 ± 0.7	7.4 ± 2.0

vealed that vasoligation resulted in reduced sperm numbers on the ligated side ($p < 0.001$) during the first 2 weeks of ligation, but there appeared to be some recovery from the second to the fifth weeks as demonstrated by a significant quadratic response with duration of ligation ($p \simeq 0.06$). In contrast, average sperm concentration on the right side showed no significant change with time. Concentration of testicular sperm was much less variable than total testicular sperm within any group of 5 rabbits, presumably because the total sperm criterion was affected by differences in the size of the rabbits and their testes. Therefore, concentration of testicular sperm is a more sensitive criterion for measurement of treatment differences.

Vasoligation reduced the number of sperm in the caput-corpus epididymides ($p < 0.05$) after 2 weeks (Table 3). But, like testicular sperm, the caput-corpus epididymidal sperm recovered to a normal number after the second week ($p < 0.01$). The weekly averages on the unligated side did not change significantly with time. In contrast to the caput-corpus epi-

212

TABLE 3. Sperm Numbers in Caput-Corpus and Cauda Epididymides after Unilateral Vasoligation ($\times 10^7$)

Duration of ligation (wk.)	Caput-corpus		Cauda		Total	
	Normal	Ligated	Normal	Ligated	Normal	Ligated
0	3.8	4.2	25.0	23.5	28.8	27.6
1	2.9	1.2	24.1	28.4	27.0	29.6
2	5.9	2.8	19.5	43.5	25.5	46.3
3	5.5	5.7	17.8	67.7	23.3	73.2
4	3.7	5.1	18.6	83.2	22.3	88.2
5	4.3	3.5	15.8	63.8	20.1	67.3
SE*	1.1	1.0	4.1	11.4	4.7	11.6

* Standard errors for N = 5.

didymides, vasoligation produced a fourfold increase in numbers of sperm in cauda epididymides ($p < 0.001$), while cauda epididymides on the unligated side exhibited a linear decline in sperm numbers with time ($p \simeq 0.07$).

When the data in Table 3 were combined, for total epididymal sperm, unilateral ligation was associated with a significant increase in epididymal sperm numbers ($p < 0.001$), while the normal side exhibited an insignificant reduction. Total epididymal sperm on the ligated side did not change appreciably during the first week of ligation, but tripled from the first to the fourth weeks and then declined to the fifth week, exhibiting a significant cubic response ($p \simeq 0.05$).

Data from rabbits after sham ligation of deferent ducts revealed no dramatic effect of this surgery. Of the seven criteria listed (Table 4), only the number of sperm in cauda epididymides 2 weeks later was significantly affected by the sham surgery ($p < 0.05$), and the dimension of this response was much smaller than the changes exhibited in the vasoligated bucks (Table 3).

DISCUSSION

Data from sham-operated bucks demonstrated that responses observed following vasoligation in the other bucks were not merely due to trauma of surgery, and consequently it was considered unnecessary to extend the sham-operational period beyond 2 weeks. Data from the sham-operated bucks and from the 0-week control group supported the conclusion that left and right halves of male rabbits' reproductive tracts do not differ appreciably.

TABLE 4. Weights and Sperm Contents of Testis and Caput-Corpus and Cauda Epididymides after Sham Ligation of Left Deferent Duct

	Weeks of ligation			
	1		2	
Criterion	Normal	Sham	Normal	Sham
Testis weight (gm.)	1.8	1.8	1.4	1.5
Sperm/gm. testis ($\times 10^7$)	12.4	10.4	12.8	12.2
Testicular sperm ($\times 10^7$)	21.6	18.6	18.4	18.0
Caput-corpus weight (gm.)	0.2	0.3	0.2	0.2
Caput-corpus sperm ($\times 10^7$)	4.6	4.9	8.8	9.4
Cauda weight (gm.)	0.4	0.4	0.4	0.4
Cauda sperm ($\times 10^7$)	18.9	20.2	30.3	34.8

Vasoligation caused a reduction in average testis weight within the first 2 weeks and cauda epididymides on the ligated side were visibly enlarged. This enlargement was linear with time of ligation, at least through 4 weeks, indicating that testicular contributions and epididymal secretions accumulated in this organ for at least 4 weeks after ligation.

Moore and Quick used histologic observations to evaluate the effects of vasectomy on spermatogenesis and concluded that vasectomy did not arrest spermatogenesis. We have also observed mitotic divisions and spermatozoa in the lumina of seminiferous tubules at all periods after vasoligation. However, these histologic observations are difficult to quantify and do not preclude the possibility that the level of spermatogenesis may have been affected. Numbers of testicular sperm are more easily quantified and provide a good estimate of level of spermatogenesis. Either total testicular sperm or sperm per gram of testicular parenchymal tissue may be used as a response criterion, but results of this experiment reveal that the latter is preferable. It is less variable, apparently, because it is not influenced by size of testis. Similarly, Almquist and Amann reported that the concentration of testicular sperm was less variable than the total in bulls.

Unilateral ligation of the deferent duct reduced testicular sperm concentration only on the ligated side. However, these changes in sperm concentration followed a quadratic response with duration of ligation, suggesting that, as with testis weight, the initial decline was followed by partial recovery. Longer intervals of ligation could have resulted in more complete recovery, because Moore and Quick reported that spermatogenesis was not disrupted even 6 months after vasectomy. These workers were critical of the results of Steinach, who suggested that vasectomy resulted in degeneration of the testis followed by a regeneration 2 weeks later. Moore and

Quick inferred that this decline in spermatogenesis and the subsequent regeneration observed by Steinach was due to temporary retention of the testis in the peritoneal cavity. In the present experiment, the rabbits were regularly examined to ascertain that the testes remained in the scrotum. Thus, our results concur with those of Steinach. However, it should be noted that the degree of response to ligation varied considerably among rabbits.

Whereas the epididymides on the vasoligated side contained increased sperm numbers, sperm numbers in the contralateral epididymides declined. On the ligated side, sperm numbers in the caput-corpus epididymides initially declined during the first week, increased from the first to the third week, and then declined again from the third to the fifth week. The initial decline was probably due to the reduction in testicular sperm at that time. However, as large numbers of sperm accumulated in the cauda epididymides, more were apparently retained in the caput-corpus region at the third week. The reduction in sperm numbers in the caput-corpus epididymidis during the final week was associated with a similar decline in the cauda epididymidis.

The greatest accumulation of sperm in the cauda epididymidis occurred 4 weeks after ligation, when sperm numbers in this organ amounted to nearly 400% of those of the controls at 0 weeks. However, in terms of sperm per gram of caudal tissue, there was only a 50% increase, suggesting that the cauda epididymidis may accommodate the increased sperm numbers by growth as well as stretching.

Superficially, the decline in total epididymal sperm from the fourth to fifth weeks of ligation seemed contradictory because it occurred at the same time that testicular sperm numbers (i.e., spermatogenesis) were returning toward normal levels. Since spermatogenesis was not arrested, the decline in total epididymidal and particularly in caudal sperm numbers was probably due to resorption of sperm from the cauda epididymides, as suggested by Orgebin-Crist. Almquist and Amann suggest that the cauda epididymidis is also the major site of sperm resorption in the bull.

The unoperated right side of the reproductive tract could not be used as a control for the ligated left side because right-side epididymal sperm numbers were not maintained at constant levels. Average sperm content of the right cauda epididymides and sperm per gram of right caudal tissue declined 37% and 57%, respectively. These declines were not associated with any significant changes in the average weight of the cauda epididymides. Since ligation of the contralateral deferent duct failed to affect testicular sperm numbers (i.e., spermatogenesis) significantly on the unoperated side, sperm must have entered the unligated epididymis at a relatively constant rate—a conclusion which is supported by data on sperm content of caput-corpus epididymides on the unligated side. Therefore, the decline in total sperm content and sperm concentration in the cauda epididymides on the unligated side was due either to increased sperm resorption at that location or to increased loss of sperm via the deferent duct.

The ratio between total epididymal sperm and total testicular sperm in sexually rested animals should reflect the sperm storage role of the epididymis relative to the supply of sperm from the testis. Changes in this ratio should reflect changes in losses of epididymal sperm, either due to resorption or via the deferent duct. The average ratios of cauda epididymidal sperm to testicular sperm on the unoperated right side (Fig. 1) declined significantly (p < 0.005) with increasing duration of ligation on the left side. A similar curve for total ratios of epididymidal to testicular sperm possessed shape (slope) nearly identical to that in Fig. 1, indicating that the decline in the ratio involving total epididymal sperm was primarily due to changes in the sperm content of the cauda epididymides.

The dramatic changes in epididymidal sperm numbers caused by ligation of the contralateral deferent duct reveal that unilateral ligation increases the loss of epididymidal sperm on the unligated side. We believe that this is the first demonstration of such an interaction between the right and left epididymides. Since sperm content of the deferent duct on the unligated side of the tract was not considered in this study, the decline in the ratios (Fig. 1) may have been due either to increased resorption of sperm from the cauda or to increased loss via the deferent duct. Immunologic assay of blood serums from similar animals for sperm-specific antibodies may help to resolve this question.

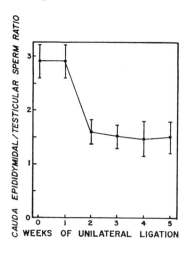

Fig. 1. Ratios of caudal epididymidal to testicular sperm on unoperated side after unilateral ligation of deferent duct. Vertical bars represent standard errors.

216

Although the curve in Fig. 1 is statistically linear ($p < 0.05$), the greatest change occurred between the first and second week after ligation. Thereafter, the declines were slight. Since there was little change in these ratios during the first week after ligation, the decreases apparent in Fig. 1 were probably not associated with surgical trauma. Rather, the large decrease in ratios of epididymidal to testicular sperm during the second week was associated with a large increase in caudal and total epididymidal sperm numbers on the ligated side. Subsequent changes in these averages on the ligated side had relatively little effect on epididymidal sperm loss on the normal side. If the ratios of epididymidal to testicular sperm had been influenced by the rate of spermatogenesis in the testis on the ligated side, the trend toward recovery of sperm numbers in this testis during the last 3 weeks should have been associated with concomitant recovery of the ratios in Fig. 1.

The data support the conclusion that when sperm content of a cauda epididymidis is increased by about 50% by unilateral vasoligation, sperm losses from the cauda epididymidis on the unligated side are dramatically increased. Further increases in sperm numbers in the epididymidis on the ligated side have little effect on sperm losses from the contralateral side.

REFERENCES

1. ALBERT, A. "The Mammalian Testis." In *Sex and Internal Secretions* (ed. 3). Young, W. C., Ed. Williams & Wilkins, Baltimore, 1961, p. 323.
2. ALMQUIST, J. O., and AMANN, R. P. Reproductive capacity of dairy bulls. II. Go-

217

nadal and extra gonadal sperm reserves as determined by direct counts and depletion trials; dimensions and weight of genitalia. *J Dairy Sci* 44:1668, 1961.

3. AMANN, R. P. Reproductive capacity of dairy bulls. III. The effect of ejaculation frequency, unilateral vasectomy, and age on spermatogenesis. *Amer J Anat 110:* 49, 1962.

4. BOUIN, P., and ANCEL, P. Recherches sur les cellules interstitielles du testicule chez les mammifères. *Arch Zool Exper Gen* 1:437, 1903.

5. KIRTON, K. T., DESJARDINS, C., and HAFS, H. D. Distribution of sperm in male rabbits after various ejaculation frequencies. *Anat Rec* 158:287, 1967.

6. MOORE, C. R., and QUICK, W. J. Properties of the gonads as controllers of somatic and psychical characteristics. VII. Vasectomy in the rabbit. *Amer J Anat* 34:317, 1924.

7. ORGEBIN-CRIST, M. C. Delayed incorporation of thymidine ³H in epithelial cells of the ductus epididymidis of the rabbit. *J Reprod Fertil* 8:259, 1964.

8. STEINACH, E. Verjungung durch experimentelle Neubelebung der altenden Pubertät sdrüse. *Wilhelm Roux'Arch Entwicklungsmech Organ* 46:557, 1920.

AUTHOR INDEX

Alderman, Phillp M., 93

Beazley, John M., 56
Bunge, R.G., 111, 198, 204

Cooke, I.D., 66
Crosby, D.L., 66

Desjardins, C., 210
Draper, John W., 190

Ferber, Andrew S., 98
Fernandes, Manuel, 190
Fraser, W.J., 56

Hafs, H.D., 210
Hancock, Carl V., 145
Hanley, Howard G., 174, 182
Henderson, William D., 145
Hershey, Nathan, 62
Horowitz, Marcel I., 146

Igboeli, G., 150

Jackson, Pauline, 66
Jones, H.O., 66

Kirton, K.T., 210

Lewit, Sarah, 98

Macmillan, K.L., 210
McGarry, J.M., 66
Mehta, K.C., 205
Moon, K.H., 111, 198

Nag, Moni, 76
Norberg, K.-A., 153

Pagovich, Benjamin L., 146
Phillips, Betson, 66

Potts, I.F., 92
Prentiss, Robert J., 10
Prosser, Elizabeth, 66
Pugh, R.C.B., 182

Rakha, A.M., 150
Ramani, P.S., 205
Rees, R.W., 66
Rinker, J. Robert, 145
Risley, Paul L., 153
Roberts, H.J., 119, 131
Rodgers, David A., 10, 30
Roe, Anne, 61
Rowson, L.E.A., 159
Rümke, Ph., 115, 120

Shah, Kanu N., 190
Skinner, J.D., 159
Smith, J.C., 55
Steinhardt, Edward E., 194

Tietze, Christopher, 98
Tindall, V.R., 66
Titus, M., 120

Ungerstedt, U., 153
Urquhart-Hay, D., 86

Watts, George, 97
Weinberg, Sidney R., 146
Wolfers, Helen, 77

Young, Donald, 96

Ziegler, Frederick J., 10, 30, 73

Abdominal Prostatectomy, 146
Abortion, 62
Adrenergic Innervation, 153

Contraception, 10, 96, 117, 172

Diabetogenic Hyperinsulinism,
   131

Epididymitis Prevention, 145

Gonadal Sperm Reserves, 210

Lacate Dehydrogenase Isozyme
   Patterns, 111
Legality, 62, 92
Long-Term Effects in Bulls,
   148

Pituitary Gonadotrophins, 150
Psychological Aspects, 10, 73,
   77, 98

Ovulation Suppressors, 30

Reanastomosis, Spontaneous,
   104; Technique for, 205
Research Proposal, 61

Semen Examinations, 55
Seminal Vesicular Fructose,
   148
Sexual Behavior, 30, 98
Sexual Development in Pubes-
   cent Mammals, 157
Sperm-Agglutinating Autoanti-
   bodies. 115
Sperm-Agglutinin Formation,
   120
Spontaneous Recanalization,
   182
Sterilization, 62, 77, 97; Vol-
   untary, 56, 86, 93, 119, 174
Sterilization Clinic, 66
Systemic Complications, 129

Techniques, 144, 188, 192, 196
Thrombophlebitis, 129

Unilateral Cryptorchism, 159

Vasovasostomy, 190, 194, 198